INCENDIARY SEX AFTER 50!

By Julia West and Michael Hart

Copyright © 2018. All Rights Reserved.

All rights reserved. No part of this book may be reproduced in any form or by any electronic or mechanical means including information storage and retrieval systems, without permission in writing from the author. The only exception is by a reviewer, who may quote short excerpts in a review.

Visit our website at www.IncendiarySex.com

Printed in the United States of America

ISBN- 9781792011542

TABLE OF CONTENTS

Incendiary Sex After 50 7
    The Best Time In Your Life is Still to Come 10
    Seniors Having Sex 13
    Who Are We? 18
    What You Will Find In This Book 23

The ABC's of Sex After 50 26
    Scheduling Sex 27
    Not Just For Bedtime, Or Even Bed 33
    Building Anticipation – Mental Foreplay 36
    Confidence 39
    Kindness 44
    His Erections 48
    You Are Not Your Penis 51
    How To Have An Erection After 50 55
    Arousal and Lubrication 59
    All About Lube 63
    Sex Toys and Orgasms 69
    Let's Visit A Sex Store 72
    What About When It Doesn't Happen 77
    Masturbation 79
    Senior VD – Yes, You Still Need Condoms 82

When It's Been A Loooong Time 85
    Breaking the Ice – How to Start the Conversation 87

 Getting In touch With Yourself 94
 Getting In Touch With Each Other 98
 Naked Time — How to Get to Great Sex by Not Having Sex. 101
 Cannabis – Take Away the Tension 103

Sex and Cannabis 104

 How to Use Cannabis In Your Love Life 106
 What to Expect the First Time 113
 Cannabis: Good or Bad? 118
 Let's Visit A Dispensary 126

How To Be Here Now 136

 Turn On the Ons, Turn Off the Offs 138
 Setting The Stage 140
 Involve All Your Senses 143
 Scents 144
 Lighting 145
 Sounds 146
 Taste 148
 Touch 149
 Warm And Clean 150
 Décor 152
 Ready and Waiting 154
 What Do I Call It? 156
 Breathing 160
 The Cannabis Ritual 162

Mating Rituals 164

 Tantra For Fun 167
 Guided Erotic Massage 175

    Better to Give or Receive? Try Both!......................... 178
    Body Mapping... 181
    Covered but Accesible.. 183
    Hot and Cold 185
    Sexy Reading.. 188
    Talk Clean To Me.. 191
    Blindfolds 194

Health 196
    Don't Believe Any of This 198
    Vaginal Dryness and Pain During Sex 199
    Erectile Difficulties 203
    Loss of Libido in Women.. 206
    Loss of Libido in Men... 213
    Sex Therapy and Counseling.. 215

Resources 216
Appendix: Erotic Guided Massage Script............................. 218
Afterword - Michael.. 233
Afterword – Julia 234

INCENDIARY SEX AFTER 50

There are those moments in everyone's life when you are "there." Remember that moment when you said "I do," and kissed? The moment when you first held your baby in your arms? The sunset you watched together with your partner, your head on his shoulder? Maybe that great tennis game when you were "on" and couldn't lose?

What do each of those moments have in common? You were "there," right there in the moment. Without a thought for the moment before or the moment after. You were living, really living with every fiber of your being. Living with everything you had.

Those are the best moments in life—what we call "Being Here Now." We can help you bring that into your love life. We are talking about those timeless moments when the world disappears and it's just the two of you sharing your bodies, your touch, your scent, your taste. Living each second fully as it happens. We are talking about toe-curling, mind-exploding white heat as you reach for a glimpse of heaven. We are talking about experiences that leave you spent and breathless and bring a happy smile and a spring to your step for the rest of the day. Incendiary sex over 50? Yes, you can have it.

You don't need a perfect body. You don't need pointy breasts or firm buttocks or an ever-ready erection. The bodies you have will do just fine. You only need to be able to create that moment where you aren't worried about what you look like or what your partner is thinking or the argument you had with your sister. You just need to Be Here Now.

We can help you with that. We show you how to temporarily take away the little pains and annoyances that come with life and age, and how to create a space made to hold those moments. We show you how to get out of your own head, how to stop the spinning dialog. We have some exercises to help that we call "Mating Rituals." But you won't need to keep a notebook to remember them, or don the scuba flippers or a spider man outfit. We aren't going to teach you new sexual positions, or complicated fantasies that include whips and handcuffs. Instead we are going to teach you how to create that space where you can be safe, naked, together, and living moment to moment. You can take it from there.

And we have one more suggestion for you to explore: legal pot. A great and slightly naughty tool to help you let go of your worries and your fears, and to stop the whirl in your head. We'll show you how to use it safely in conjunction with all of our other tools to enhance your love life.

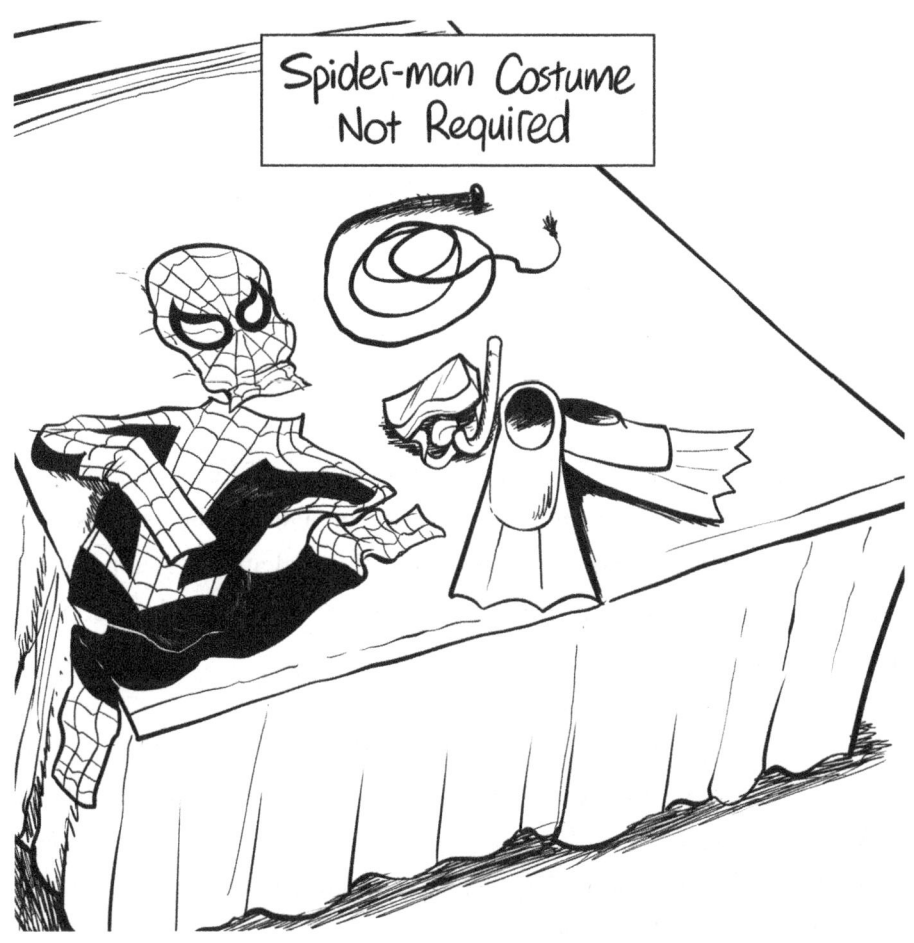

Maybe it's been a loooong time for you. Maybe there is a lot of tension and baggage to get through. We will try to help you find a path back to each other. Whether you are in your 60s, 70s, 80s or more, you have all you need to have a close, loving, sensual time, and perhaps find the best loving you've ever had in your life. Come on the journey with us, and begin to make your life better.

THE BEST TIME IN YOUR LIFE IS STILL TO COME

These are truly your Golden Years. This is not just a pretty platitude to distract you from the fact that you are losing your hair and your hearing. It's the truth. From age 50 on, as dozens of studies show, the older you get, the happier you are. For many of us, the best times of our lives are still to come.

According to a study from the London School of Economics which looked at several categories of "happiness," on average the happiest age is 69, while people's happiness with their physical appearance peaks in their 70s and 80s. Overall life satisfaction was the highest between the ages of 82 and 85.

A University of Chicago study based on periodic face-to-face interviews with 28,000 people from 18 to 88 years old found that the odds of being happy increased five percent with every 10 years of age after 50.[1] As study author Yang Yang summarized: "The good news is that with age comes happiness."

A 2016 study of adults aged 21 to 99 published in the journal Psychology and Aging found that, on average, mental well-being steadily improved as people grew older, despite the fact that older adults had more physical health issues and problems with memory and

---

[1] https://news.uchicago.edu/story/age-comes-happiness-university-chicago-study-shows

cognition than younger people.[2] The study found happiness ratings rising gradually and steadily from age 50 through the decade of the 90s.

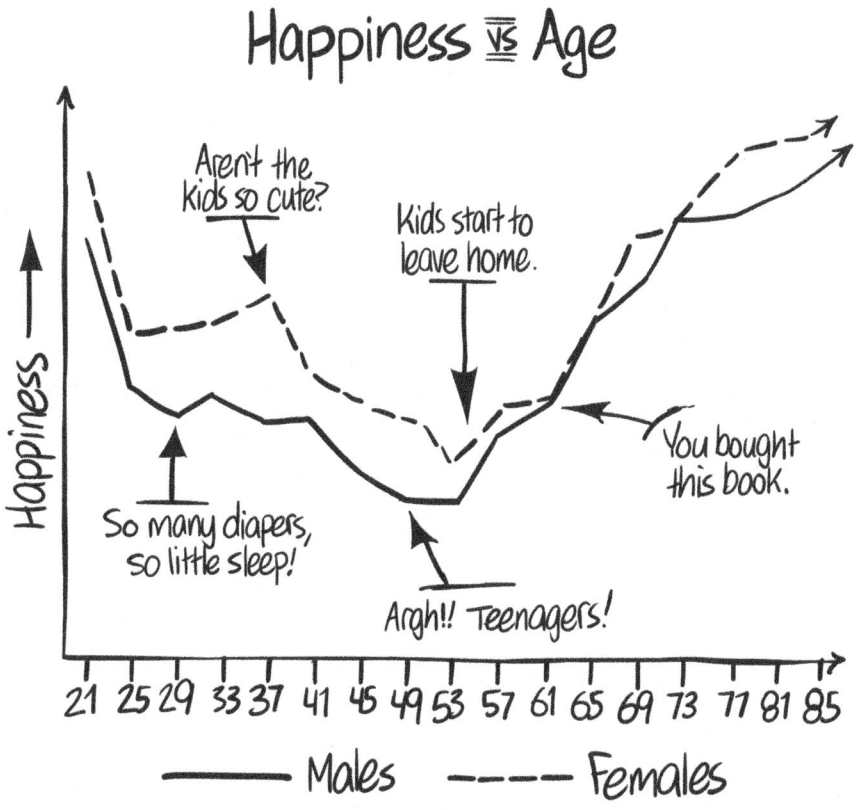

Given the common well-known problems associated with aging, why this growing happiness as the years tick by? There appear to be several reasons. Some study authors point to seniors having better wisdom on

---

[2] http://www.latimes.com/science/sciencenow/la-sci-sn-older-people-happier-20160824-snap-story.html

how to cope with life's ups and downs. Better emotional stability, say others. Seniors tend to invest in what is most important to them, often focusing on savoring close relationships and on emotionally meaningful goals and activities.

There is a wisdom and clearer perspective that comes to those of us who have more miles on our odometers than are left on our warranties. After all, why not be optimistic? Don't we have what we've always wanted as teenagers, just several decades late? You don't have to go to school, or maybe even work. You get an allowance every month. You have your own car. You have your own pad, no curfew, and a driver's license that gets you into bars and legal pot dispensaries. And you can have hotter sex than you did when you were a teenager without worrying about getting pregnant.

SENIORS HAVING SEX

As we noted above, most of us are or will be happier in our 60s, 70s and 80s than we ever were in our 30s and 40s. Many seniors who are in relationships are still having and enjoying sexual pleasure into their 70s, 80s, and even beyond. Unfortunately this isn't always the case, however. Some of the reasons that we stop having sex are because our bodies are changing, and we have not known ways of adapting to the changes. This is one place where we hope to help.

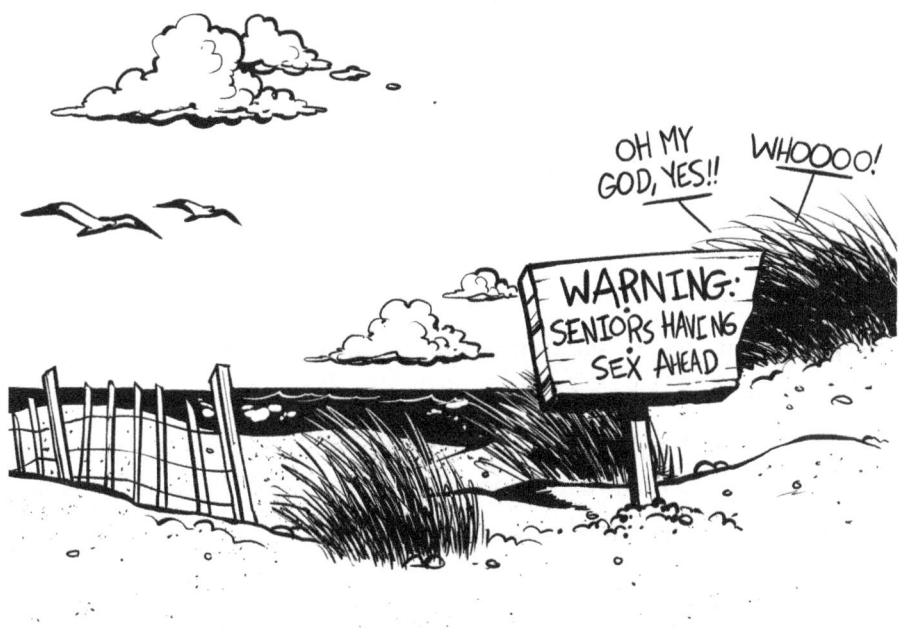

Seniors are having sex, and most are not too shy to talk about it. In a recent University of Manchester study of over 7,000 seniors that included detailed questions on their sex lives, only three percent of the respondents declined to answer these personal questions.[3] The study found that 54 percent of men and 31 percent of women over the age of 70 were still sexually active, with a third saying they had sex at least twice a month.

This complements an earlier 2007 study reported in the New England Journal of Medicine which found that while sexual activity does decline with age, a significant number of men and women reported engaging in intercourse, oral sex and/or masturbation even into their 80s and 90s.[4] Of the 3,005 men and women in this study, 73 percent of the respondents between 57 and 64 years of age were still sexually active, as were 53 percent of those aged 65 to 74, and even 26 percent of those aged 75 to 85.

Not only are seniors having sex, but many say they enjoy sex more now than when they were younger, which proves that incendiary sex doesn't require a taut body or bouncy breasts. In a study by the National Commission on Aging (NCOA), 62 percent of women over 70 reported finding sex "at least as satisfying or more satisfying physically" than it was in their 40s.[5] The study also reported that both men and women found sex in their senior years more emotionally satisfying. However, the study also reported that 40 percent of men over 70 say they would like more sex. Again, maybe we can help.

Need more reasons to have more and better sex?

---

[3] https://www.huffingtonpost.com/lifetime-daily/sex-and-seniors-whats-nor_b_14226416.html
[4] https://www.nejm.org/doi/full/10.1056/NEJMoa067423
[5] https://www.thedailybeast.com/sex-and-the-senior-citizen-how-the-elderly-get-it-on

Sex promotes vaginal health. Vaginal health depends on sexual activity. After menopause, the lack of estrogen causes women's vaginas to dry up, which can lead to vaginal atrophy and painful sex. Sex, including masturbation, keeps your vaginal walls moist and supple, and helps the body to create more lubrication. This will aid in avoiding the risk of pain or tearing.

Sex promotes a healthy heart. Sex increases blood flow and improves cardiovascular fitness and helps us maintain our strength and flexibility.

Sex can reduce pain. Relief from pain can be a side effect of sexual activity, and can't we all use a little less pain? People have reported a decrease in headaches and arthritis pain after sex. Sex produces the hormone oxytocin, leading to an increase in endorphins, which can make us feel better both emotionally and physically.

Having sex can reduce your chances of erectile dysfunction. This is a case of "use it or lose it." A study in the American Journal of Medicine with 989 men aged 55 to 75 found that prolonged abstinence promoted erectile dysfunction, and that men having sex once a week or more have only half the risk of erectile dysfunction as those that have little or no regular sex.[6]

Sex increases the emotional connection with your partner. Coming together (or even separately, pun intended), with intimate touching and

---

[6] http://www.foxnews.com/story/2008/10/23/foxsexpert-senior-sex-use-it-or-lose-it.html

loving gives us a sense of emotional well-being that can enhance our lives.

Of course, sex has never been without risk. Venereal disease, VD for short, is almost as common among the 60-and-over crowd as it is among 20-somethings. The difference is that the 20-somethings have been brought up on a steady diet of information on safe sex, which wasn't as prevalent when we were young. Singles in their 60s have lower rates of condom use than any group. This lack of awareness about safe sex, new widows and widowers who may be looking for partners after decades of monogamy, and friendly (perhaps too friendly?) retirement communities, have resulted in rising rates of VD among seniors, with the occurrence of syphilis alone up 52 percent since 2007. If you are a sexually active single, take this seriously. See our section on "Senior VD" for more information.

Our healthcare system seems to be catching up with this unfortunate trend. In 2012, Medicare began providing free annual screenings for senior citizens for chlamydia, gonorrhea, and syphilis. Someone was thinking of us!

However, while many older men and women are enjoying regular sex, too many have stopped, and half of the seniors who are sexually active report having at least one serious sexual problem. The most common of these problems include:

- Low sexual desire in women
- Difficulty with vaginal lubrication
- Inability to orgasm for women and men

- Painful intercourse for women
- Erectile difficulties for men
- Performance anxiety for men and women
- Major health issues such as diabetes and heart disease

Aside from some major health issues, the good news is that for many men and women there are solutions to these problems, many of which can be found in our "Health" section. With love, respect, a few helpful hints, and a willingness to bring sex back into your relationship, you and your partner could move into the "Yes!" or even the "Oh My God, Yes!!" column.

WHO ARE WE?

We are not professional sex therapists or licensed psychologists. We are a middle-aged couple who want to keep the passion and heat—and the emotional connection that comes with it—to the very end of our lives (or at least damn close). Michael and Julia are our pen names, not our real names, as our children are unlikely to want to hear about their dad's erections or their mother's favorite sex toys and mating rituals. Nor do we think our professional associates will want to know about this intimate side of us.

We met in our 40s and we had a hot connection from the start. Our early days together had plenty of sleepless but memorable nights, and for the first year we practically needed a board down the middle of the bed to get some sleep, as just a single touch could send us off again.

That early white-hot love faded somewhat over time. However, both of us believed in the importance of keeping a strong intimate relationship, and worked to make it a priority in our lives. But as the years went by, we noticed that what used to work for us really didn't anymore.

First, we noticed that while we still had great sex on vacations or away from the house, it was harder and harder to get into the mood while at home. And as the kids got older and more time passed, we began to see changes in ourselves. Michael began to suffer the occasional out-of-service day, which was a surprise and brought with it all the attendant worries a guy has about that. And as Julia went through menopause, she found her drive for sex changing, and found orgasms often harder and harder to reach.

Luckily, we cared about each other and our love life, and worked to find ways of keeping alive the passion that we loved so much. We'd both had prior relationships in which the romance had died completely, and knew first-hand that when the passion and romance is gone, the soul of the relationship suffers as well. Initially, we assumed the issue was relaxation, contrasting the relaxation of vacations or stay-cations to the chaos of our regular lives at home. Upon further exploration, we came to find ways to create distraction from the mental chatter that was preventing us from connecting and staying present. We worked on finding ways to take away the worries of the day and focus on each other. Through trial and error, we began to collect a set of tools to keep our love life alive: oils and toys, books, candles and little "mating rituals" that we invented and enjoyed together.

> *When the passion and romance is gone, the soul of the relationship suffers as well*

Finally, after years of experimentation we slowly came to realize what was at the bottom of not only the very best sexual times in our lives, but the very best times in our lives period: We started to learn how to "Be Here Now." How to live and enjoy the moment, to savor life as it comes, second by second, without reference to future or past. To really be together, now.

Our bodies and minds were changing as we went through this journey, but even with these changes we found that our new understanding, along with the growing bucket of "tools" we had at our disposal, were not just keeping our sex life alive, but giving us a sex life that was better than ever—on its best days somewhere between insanely glorious and godlike.

And then something new came to our state: legal pot. While Michael had been an extremely casual user over the years, sometimes going decades without, Julia had only a few college experiences with cannabis, and both of us were a little nervous about reaching out for something that had been illegal our entire lives.

What we found to our delight was a new tool for our arsenal to create that ability to "Be Here Now." One that could help us stop the spinning in our heads and enjoy those amazing moments where the rest of the world disappears, and we are really living right here, right now.

Not that learning about pot after all those years didn't have a few glitches. We got too high a few times, we tried stuff that actually turned off our sex drive, and we woke up still stoned in the middle of the night after eating edibles.

But in the end, we found that the judicious use of legal pot—this new fun and somewhat naughty tool—along with the suite of tools we had already developed in working to keep our love life alive, was giving us something that none of our friends or acquaintances seemed to have: a strong love life that included absolutely white-hot, over-the-line, incendiary sex.

We decided to share what we had learned, to bring to others the joy that we had discovered in our lives. We wanted to help give others the thrill of knowing that, despite aging bodies, the best time in your life may still be to come, and even the best sex in your life may still be to come.

We are very accepting people, and we know that there is a spectrum of different gender identities, sexual interests, and types of relationships. Our own kids have stretched our understanding of gender and sex. Among our wonderful children we have those who identify as heterosexual, bisexual, pansexual and transgender, and we recognize that a more comprehensive book could be written with all of these particular concerns and challenges in mind. We know that there are many challenges to a healthy sex life for single or widowed men and women, those with severe health problems, weight problems, addiction issues and more that we have not covered fully. However, we can only write about what we know. We are two older, married, heterosexual Americans living in a state that now has legal cannabis. We hope that the tools we have developed for a happier sexier life can help many other people, regardless of situation or orientation. Take what we have to offer and adapt as needed!

Join us on the journey, and learn how to Be Here Now.

[**Julia**] *I was married for 14 years to the father of my children. While the very early days of our relationship were sexy and happy, our love life pretty quickly took a turn to dullsville with the transition to parenthood, busy work lives, and the like. I quite simply lost all desire.*

I started playing little tricks like undressing for bed in the closet or bathroom so that I would not inadvertently arouse my husband. I withheld passionate goodnight kisses for fear of sending a signal that I was game for some fun that night. After years of this sexual distance, I found myself wondering if I was simply broken or dead inside.

Now fast forward three years post-divorce to my second date with Michael. I remember so clearly sitting on the couch in my living room and talking with him after a wonderful dinner at a cozy restaurant. He subconsciously started playing with my hair as we were talking. He suddenly caught himself and asked me if what he was doing was alright. Alright? Little did he know that playing with my hair was one of my magic buttons. I'll spare you the details, but let's just say that the night ended with him scooping me up in his arms, carrying me upstairs to my bedroom and me suddenly realizing that I was neither dead inside nor broken. All systems were most definitely a "Go!"

I tell you this story because I think my experience is actually quite common. Over time, many people become comfortable with a growing distance between themselves and their partner, and they make an assumption that they really just don't need or want sex anymore—or worse—that they aren't really even capable of enjoying it. What I learned loud and clearly that night (and on many nights thereafter!) is that our bodies can be dormant for a long time, but that does not mean they are closed for business. With time, patience, some experimentation and the right combination of physical and emotional chemistry, you might just be amazed at what that ol' body is capable of. Here's hoping your surprises are as happy as mine were!

WHAT YOU WILL FIND IN THIS BOOK

OK, so now you know that the best part of your life is still to come, that seniors in their 60s, 70s, and 80s can and do have satisfying sex, and you've learned a bit about Michael and Julia, your authors. (That's assuming that you didn't just skip right to this section. If you did, go back and read from the start. It's inspiring!). We have sprinkled insights and useful tips throughout this book, but in general here is what you will find in the various sections of the book:

- The ABC's of Sex After 50. One thing is true and can't be avoided: sex is different as we age, and what used to work for us before may not now. In "The ABCs of Sex After 50," we'll show you solutions to the changes in our bodies and our psychology that are interfering with a great sex life. We will show you how scheduling sex, which might sound to you like the least sexy thing, may be the key to bringing back your sex life. We'll talk about building anticipation, and how confidence and kindness together create the environment where romance can flourish. We'll talk about the realities of erections, arousal and lubrication at our age, about the magic of sex toys, what to do when things just aren't working, masturbation and even Senior VD.

- When It's Been a Loooong Time. If your answer to the question "When was the last time you had good sex?" is "What year is it now, anyway?", then maybe you need to read these sections. Nothing has more emotional baggage attached to it than sex. We'll show you how to have the conversations that will lead you back to each other. We'll show you how to calm your fears and how you can help your partner calm theirs. We will show you strategies to help ease you back into actually being together naked, how to reconnect with your body, and tips on how a little legal pot can turn your tension, fears and worries into laughter.

- Sex and Cannabis. While tips on using pot as a tool to help your sex life are sprinkled throughout the book, here is where we'll give you the real low-down. If you've never used marijuana, or your last toke on a joint was 1978, then you'll enjoy a head-spinning introduction into the new world of legal pot and all the advice you need to get started. Even if you've partaken now and then over the years, we'll give you the tips you need to use cannabis to help ignite your sex life. This isn't about getting high; it's about stopping the spinning in your head and helping you reach that "Be Here Now" moment. Much of the advice you will get at your local pot dispensary can lead you astray when it comes to using pot judiciously to juice up the romance, so even if you think you know about cannabis, don't miss this section!

- How to Be Here Now. The key to incendiary sex is to "Be Here Now," where you are living the moment without reference to the future, past, or the thousand chores spinning in your head. In our smart-phone, media-streaming world you may need some help to get there. We will show you how to "Turn On the Ons, and Turn Off the Offs," and help you create the perfect environment to find those moments.

You'll learn how breathing and perhaps a little pot can help ease the last of the tension, and you may even learn a few new names for your and your partner's genitalia that won't make you cringe when you hear them.

- <u>Mating Rituals</u>. Here we put the "play" back into "foreplay," with games that don't require hand cuffs, complicated rules or scuba flippers. You won't find diagrams of new sex positions here, but you will find personally tested and approved playtime activities that have led us to countless orgasms and mind-blowing incendiary sex sessions.

- <u>Health</u>. Even if the spirit is willing, the flesh may be weak. Erection difficulties, loss of libido, problems with arousal, lubrication and pain during sex can make "Being Here Now" difficult or impossible. The good news is that in almost all cases, there are solutions to your problems, many of which you may not know about.

- <u>All The Rest</u>. At the end of this book you will also find sex and sexual-health related resources, as well as our personally tested and orgasmically approved Erotic Guided Massage Script.

THE ABC'S OF SEX AFTER 50

You've gained your freedom. Your kids are out of the house, and there is nobody to complain about you and your partner making out in the kitchen. No one to see you walk around the house half undressed. No one to hear your moans emanating from the bedroom. Gone are the days of shuttling kids to soccer games and school events. Maybe you aren't even working full time anymore. Isn't this kind of freedom what you could only dream about when you were 30? With all this privacy and free time, this could be the most steamy and passionate time of your life. But is it?

Probably not. After all, you're reading this book! Maybe menopause has put a "pause" in your love life. Maybe you're embarrassed about your aging body, or occasional erection troubles. Perhaps sex has begun to feel painful, or your arthritis pain keeps pricking you during lovemaking. Maybe with the kids gone, you find you have a hard time coming up with anything to talk about except, well, the kids. Perhaps you are just bored with sex, which hasn't changed much for you in the last 20 years, and what used to work for you just doesn't seem to work any more.

The good news is that all your troubles have solutions, and that with all this privacy, free time, and the sexual "tools" you can find here, this really can be the most steamy, passionate time of your life.

SCHEDULING SEX

While our bodies are changing, our attitudes about sex often don't change. Shouldn't sex be spontaneous? That overwhelming feeling that comes over us, causing us to start tearing off each other's clothes as prelude to a passionate, breathless and often short sex scene?

That was honeymoon sex. Young love sex. And it probably worked for many years after, at least now and then. But as the years passed, have you found that those blinding moments of passion happened less and less? How often does that happen now? Can you think back to the last time it happened?

If your answer to the last question is "What year is it now?" you are not alone. You may find, particularly if you are a woman, that while you enjoy sex when it happens, you can go for days or weeks where it hardly passes your mind. If so, you are in the majority of senior citizens. As a post-menopausal woman, the biological drive that you had to procreate is gone. Without the need to lure a mate and fill a womb, the hormones that spurred you to the peak of spontaneous passion are no longer needed, and so your body is not producing them.

You want sex and passion, but your body has changed, and what worked before not only won't work now, but would not be as good for you or as satisfying if it did. You take longer than you used to to get excited and lubricate, and you need that lubrication more, as your vaginal walls have thinned, and sex without sufficient foreplay could be painful, even damaging. You may not climax as quickly, and so a rapid thrusting is not likely to be as satisfying as you may have once found it.

The answer to this dwindling level of spontaneous desire is to *schedule sex*. What may sound to your ears like the least romantic thing possible may be just the thing to put more romance back into your life.

We schedule important things, don't we? Special dinners with family, vacations, events with the kids. Scheduling a special time to be together tells your partner how important they are to you, and how much you value your sex life together. If an intimate life with your partner is important to you, why not show it by putting sex ahead of fertilizing the lawn, cleaning out the refrigerator, and the thousand other things on your mind?

But the best part of scheduling sex is the anticipation. Foreplay starts with setting a time, a Date Night. The thought of the special evening or lazy afternoon to come begins the process of putting your mind in the mood.

Scheduling a sex date allows you to prepare, and to create the environment and conditions that make good loving more likely to happen. Please see "How to Be Here Now" for tips on how to create the space to be in the moment. We won't repeat these tips in this section, but here are a few general themes that will help you make this a success.

One idea is to make the sex just one part of a fun evening. Cook up a meal together while drinking wine. Maybe play a fun game that gets you invigorated. Any activity that's fun, light and playful makes it easy to segue into foreplay. You can build up to the event over days, building anticipation. Just a little text "I'm thinking of being with you tomorrow night" can start the juices flowing.

Of course if you haven't had sex in a while, or it has been very sporadic, scheduling sex can cause stress and worry over performance as the time grows near. See "It's Been a Loooong Time" for tips on bringing romance and sex back into your life after a long hiatus. One way to reduce the stress is to take baby steps. Make it clear from the start that there is no expectation of actual intercourse, just that you spend an hour naked and warm together, and "see how it goes." You may even want to affirmatively take having sex off the table to make sure you both feel comfortable getting close again without that extra stress and pressure of going "all the way." Even if you only end up with a naked backrub, it's brought you closer together emotionally, and made sex in the future more likely. What do you have to lose? An hour spent naked with your lover adds an hour to your life.

An hour spent naked with your lover adds an hour to your life.

Some people live by schedules, and find a set date at 3 p.m. every Saturday or 6 p.m. Tuesdays allows them to plan their week but enjoy the happy anticipation of upcoming liaisons. Others find the rigid regularity to be stressful in itself. In any case, you need some loving flexibility put into whatever plan you decide on. For us, scheduling sex is more of a matter of just planning for it a few days ahead. "Honey, I'd really like to spend some time together. Tomorrow's bad because of that dinner meeting, but what do you think about making time Thursday?" Other couples may find that scheduling with variation keeps things fresh. "Mutual Masturbation Mondays" anyone?

Once in a while it just won't work, regardless of mutual interest and good planning. On those occasions, you need to let it go, and not make anyone the bad guy or gal. You might be disappointed in missing something that you looked forward to, but just reschedule for another day. Getting huffy about it will only add stress to your next session.

In bringing up this idea to your partner or spouse, be sure to do it in a way that isn't accusatory or that puts them on the defensive. "We never have sex, and I think the only way we ever will is to schedule it" is probably the wrong approach. Something like, "Hey my love, I know that I've been so busy that I haven't been making enough time for you and me. I'm sorry. Can we make sure to keep this Sunday free for some you and me time?," may go down better.

Scheduling sex can also help solve a common conflict: who initiates sex. If one person is always doing the initiating, that person can feel hurt. "I always want her. Why doesn't she want me back? Doesn't she love me?" By scheduling sex, you've made a mutual agreement, one that shows both parties want to spend more intimate and romantic time together.

You may find that scheduling time for sex actually creates more spontaneous sex. Having sex leads to more sex. Reminding your body about sex puts more thoughts of sex into your mind, which can create the mood for sex regardless of the date.

Don't stop with scheduling sex. Anything that helps your love and relationship is worth taking the effort to plan for. Schedule that hike, or a plan to watch that movie, or to enjoy that lovely meal out. No matter how much Julia and I love sex with each other, it's only one part of a loving relationship.

Finally, scheduling sex and taking the time to create the space and environment for it to happen takes effort. Be sure to thank your partner, and let them know how it made you feel that they cared enough to help make this happen.

NOT JUST FOR BEDTIME, OR EVEN BED

Do you have just one time of the day when you make love? Perhaps right before you go to sleep after a full day? If that works well for you, great. But many people find that timing is everything, and as our bodies change that timing changes, and we need to adapt to it. Plus, as the famous Dr. Ruth says: "Boredom is a lot more dangerous to a relationship than any other factor," so why not mix it up a bit and see what happens?

> *"Boredom is a lot more dangerous to a relationship than any other factor." – Dr. Ruth Westheimer.*

First, timing is everything. Evening sex can be wonderful and of course has the advantage that you can lay back, spent and sexually satisfied, and just drift off to happy dreams. However, by evening your body may be in the middle of a shut-down process readying itself for sleep, and asking your body to switch from shut-down to overdrive may be asking too much. You just may not have enough energy. Try a lazy afternoon delight. If you are retired, an afternoon romp followed by an afternoon nap can be heavenly. Just ask us! Many studies show that a man's testosterone actually peaks in the morning, and he may find that he has more energy and less erection trouble in the a.m..

Plus, there are certain times of the day that you will have more energy than other times. Learn this about yourself, and put what you've learned into practice. Lovers with arthritis often find that their arthritis hurts less during certain times of the day, or perhaps within a certain time window after taking medication. Arthritis shouldn't be a barrier to sex, it should be a reason to have sex! Aside from helping with general flexibility, the hormones released during sex reduce pain, as does the legal pot we suggest you try as an aid to "Being Here Now." After all, pain relief is why millions of people use medicinal marijuana, and why it's legal in 30 States and Canada, despite strong opposition.

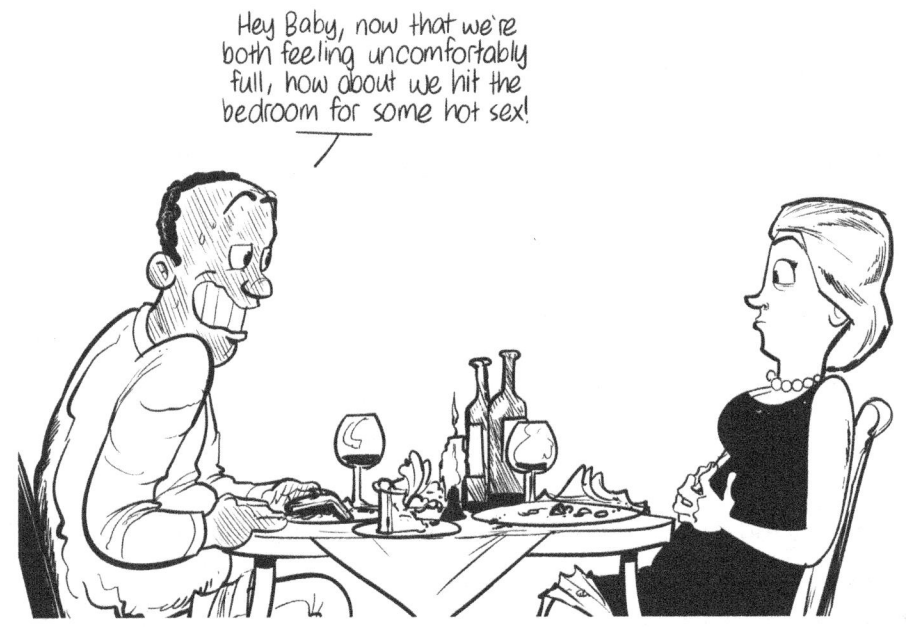

Oh, and watch out for the "Romantic Dinner." Unfortunately, this is a bit of an oxymoron. Of course, taking your lover out for a wonderful meal is a very romantic thing to do, but a bloated, gassy stomach from heavy, rich food and alcohol is not conducive to a hot night of incendiary sex. Also, both erections and female arousal depend on blood flow. (See "Her Lubrication" and "How to Have an Erection After 50.") If your body is working hard to digest a big dinner it doesn't always have blood flow to spare for your nether regions. Make love before dinner, or have a light snack, a round of insanely hot sex, and then a gorgeous dessert—preferably with chocolate! You'll think it never tasted so great.

And bed? Bed is a great place to have sex, absolutely. However, having sex outside of bed has many advantages. It's a little naughty, after all, you wouldn't dare do this when the kids where home, would you? Also, if your bedroom is where you've made love a thousand times, but also had a few terrible arguments, then this emotional baggage can intrude on the sensual and in-the-moment romantic atmosphere you are going for. Make love on the couch, in the spare bedroom, in front of the fireplace, or even propped up on the kitchen counter. Do your bones ache at the thought of laying out on a hard surface? No problem. Lay down some thick blankets or buy that sheepskin rug. Imagine two naked bodies, entwined on the floor and warmed by the flickering firelight. That could be you.

At our age it's easy to be a curmudgeon. "It'll be too hard," you might say, or, "that's just stupid," if you're a *real* curmudgeon. If you want great sex, you need to change your attitude. If your lover wants to do something new, give it a try. Asking for sex, or asking for something new with sex is a very vulnerable thing to do. If you care for your lover, don't shut your lover down when they suggest something new. Give it a whirl. What do you have to lose? If you don't like it, just strike it off the list. If you do like it, your partner will be beaming and proud for having created a new adventure, and you'll be happier. Don't be the curmudgeon. Give it a try.

BUILDING ANTICIPATION – MENTAL FOREPLAY

It's Tuesday, and you've both agreed to do whatever you need to do to make time for a Thursday night rendezvous. The lovemaking doesn't start on Thursday evening. It starts now. Building that sexual tension and anticipation will not only make a great sex session more likely, but it creates that emotional connection that many women need. Many women need to feel that emotional closeness to be able respond physically and sexually. And while guys tend to be physical first and emotional second, most guys will still enjoy an extended mental "tease."

Whisper something naughty in your partner's ear and then walk away. Text little flirty messages during the day. Some people find explicit dirty talk a turn on, detailing every little thing you are going to do to each other. Know your partner, however. Many people are shut down by crude references. (See our section on "What Do I Call It?") It may be safer to stick with simple messages like "Thinking about tomorrow night, Hot Stuff. Yummm…" or "I've got something planned for tomorrow, and I've got a feeling you're going to like it."

Get a bit touchy-feely, "accidently" brushing against your partner in a place they like, even in public if no one is watching. Grab your partner for a quick but passionate kiss.

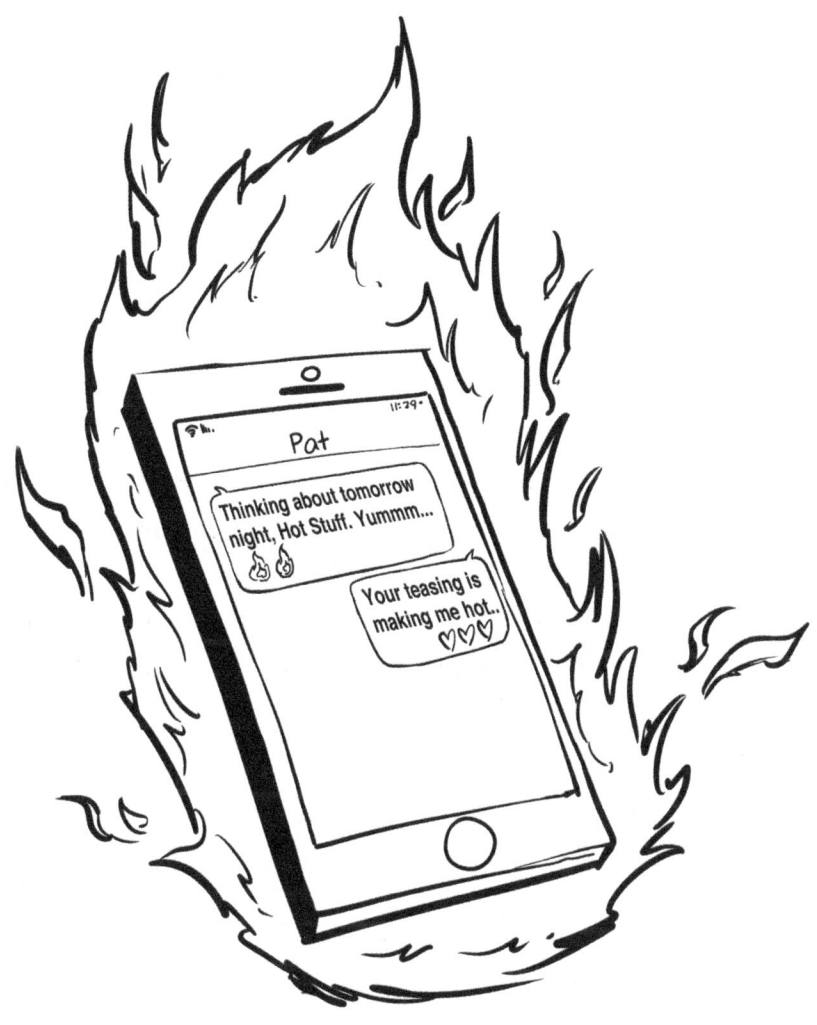

[Michael] *It doesn't have to be sexual touching. I casually massage the back of Julia's neck, or play with the little ringlets of her hair. This has become such a habit that I do it automatically without realizing it, like when we are sitting together watching TV. My wife thinks she's a*

lucky woman to have me touch her like that, and then later makes sure that I feel like a lucky guy.

With the changes in our bodies and minds that happen as we age, we need more reminding of our sexuality and a longer time to build up. Mental foreplay will make each of you feel loved and wanted. And building a broad base of sexual energy makes for a bigger peak of incendiary passion.

[Julia] *I think a lot of women want to feel seen and desired as whole people, not just sexual playthings. To that end, foreplay can include taking the time to notice and help with little things that might make your partner's life easier, like unloading the dishwasher or putting away that basket of laundry. These little niceties show your partner you love and appreciate all she does. Remember, women want to make love when they are feeling loved.*

CONFIDENCE

You've heard confident people are considered attractive and sexy by others? Well, it's true. But more importantly, confidence makes *you* want to be with you. There is no better way into a partner's heart and underwear than to lose your self-consciousness and be happy in your own body. If you're not worried about the way your belly or breasts look, if you're not worried about the visible rolls that show when you sit a certain way, then it's easier for your partner to live within their body as well, and that's when the fun can begin. Lose that distracting voice in your head "Does he like the way I look?," "Am I making a funny face?," "Does she like what I'm doing right now?" Ease out of your spinning mind and enjoy the sensations, touch, taste, and scent of the person you're with. Live second to second, and notice how your partner's body responds to you and how your body responds to their body. Notice, respond, notice, respond, notice, respond, and soon you are on a positive spiral that builds and builds until…

Well, you get the picture. Easier said than done, you say? Sure. Everyone, no matter how confident they seem, loses it now and then, and if you've been a self-loathing addict for years, it can take time to reprogram your mind. It's like gardening: you need to water and feed your self-love every day. Pull the weeds that choke out your self-love (and you might have a nasty patch of weeds in your garden to start). When you are happy within yourself and your body, you can have fun—real fun—in lovemaking. Here is a truth that you should remember: There is no greater gift you can give your partner than to have a really good time. If you have fun, your partner is going to have fun. That's not selfish, it's just the truth that you can't give away what you don't have.

> *There is no greater gift you can give your partner than to have a really good time. If you have fun, your partner is going to have fun.*

Being confident in yourself has nothing to do with having a hot, youthful body like the ones you see paraded in front of you every time you turn on the TV. (And what is it about those detective shows, where every detective is 26 years old and straight off a supermodel shoot? Really??). It has to do with loving yourself, the body you're living in and the person you are. If your partner wants to get naked with you, they are attracted to you, all of you. Let it go. Amy Schumer is a good role model. As she said at her acceptance speech at the Glamour Awards, "I'm 160 pounds, and I can catch a dick whenever I want."

> *"I'm 160 pounds, and I can catch a dick whenever I want."*
> *Amy Schumer – Glamour Awards Acceptance Speech*

How can you break a lifetime of self-loathing? How can you forget some horrible thing an ex-spouse said? How can you stop spectating in your mind when making love, and just live in the present? Here are a few tips that you may want to start living today, and everyday:

Complement your appearance, every single day. You have a nice smile. Love the toes. Great eyebrows. Great style. Lovely calves. If you are the type who can't stand to look at yourself in the mirror, get over it. Love the real you. Love the real you and your partner will too.

When thinking about your body, don't just think of it in terms of its physical appearance. Think of all the amazing things your body can do. These arms help me hug my grandchild. My legs take me for beautiful walks. My heart beats in perfect rhythm without any effort on my part. If you really stop to take in all the ways in which your various systems work in harmony every second of every day it is hard to feel distasteful toward this incredible machine.

Give a compliment to YOU, as a person, every single day. You're a good listener. You're a caring friend. You keep a wonderful house. You cook a mean turkey. You're a great mom. You might even try writing these down each night before you go to bed. There is a significant and growing body of evidence to prove that variations of this kind of Gratitude journaling can have dramatic effects on your mental health and self-esteem.

Speak to yourself like you would your children. If you have kids, do you continually point out the acne, or the weird nose, or say, "My aren't you homely?" Of course you don't. You fill them with compliments, inspiration and love for themselves and the gifts they have. You do this because you love them and want them to have a strong self-worth, so that they can be the best people they can be. Should you do less for yourself?

Imagine it all going wrong. Sounds counterintuitive? Not so. Think about what you might do in bed: spill the lube, elbow in the face, not able to get an erection, poke her uncomfortably. Now, think of the suave and smooth ways that you'll laugh together about it, get past all that and back to the fun.

Laughter. This is definitely part of the "imagine it all going wrong" bit. Laughing with, rather than at, yourself or your partner when something goes awry will relieve the tension, keep things positive, and help both of you feel happy and connected.

Don't sweat the erection. This is a big one (pun intended). If you are a man, read "You Are Not Your Penis." If you are a woman, know that even when working well, erections for an older man often wax and wane throughout lovemaking. And if things are just not working, it is NOT because "he can't be excited because I don't look good enough." He may stammer something like "Honey, it's really not you." You know what? *It's Really Not You.* He got naked with you because he was attracted to you. Read "His Erection,"—please.

Dress up. If a little make up and that hot little dress makes you feel good, put it on! Take ten minutes to make yourself feel like, "You don't have to tell me I'm beautiful. I am beautiful." Also, you may find lingerie to be silly, but if your partner buys you some, it's because he finds you sexy and wants to see you in it. Put it on and strike a sexy pose.

Better posture. Stand up straight when you walk. Put those shoulders back. Take up space. Strut, Baby. Here's the truth: your body tells you how to feel. Dozens of studies have proven this. If you force yourself to smile, you feel happier. If you walk like you own it all, you feel more confident.

Masturbate. Make your body feel good just because, and in the process learn more about your body and what you enjoy, and build up the inner juices that will make lovemaking better.

Fake it 'til you make it. We are talking confidence here, not orgasms! If you act confident, you'll feel confident. People will be attracted to you, and you'll feel even better. This is a positive spiral. The truth is that no matter how confident a person seems, there are times they are faking it.

Remember, it's like a garden. Water your sense of self-worth every single day, and soon you'll be in the moment, knowing nothing but the sensations that you and your partner are making together. Incendiary, Baby.

KINDNESS

Do you want to spark your love life into full blown incendiary sex? Then the first, best, and always necessary feature to add to your relationship is kindness. Kindness is the bedrock upon which you can build a mountain of satisfying climaxes.

The key to some of the best sex of your lives is your ability to "Be Here Now," to enjoy the moment and only the moment, with your whole world revolving around the touch, taste and scent of your partner, and your body's reaction to theirs. To reach these moments of shared intimacy, we need to feel emotionally safe and secure, and to feel emotionally safe, we need kindness.

"Being Here Now" is intimate. It can make a person feel vulnerable, exposed, scary, risky, and a single thoughtless comment can ruin the trust that you've built. While there are many myths about men's indiscriminate readiness for sex, a man is unlikely to be ready for this level of intimacy if he feels criticized, disapproved of and unappreciated by his partner. Conversely, women need to feel loved, cherished and appreciated first, before their sexual impulses are activated.

Both men and women want and need to be regarded favorably by their partners. You won't reach the intimacy required for great sex if either partner feels disregarded, shamed, criticized or diminished. It's hard to feel loving toward a partner who is harsh and disapproving.

Kindness comes from the heart and is protective of your partner. You don't want them to suffer, to be hurt, embarrassed, or diminished in any way. You go out of your way to preserve your partner's dignity and esteem. You minimize the impact of their mistakes. You find ways of making them feel valued, and show them that you appreciate them for who they are. Feeling valued is an aphrodisiac. To be intimate, we need to feel appreciated and accepted for who we are. I am sure that you realize this about yourself. Did you realize that it's true for your partner as well?

> ***Feeling valued is an aphrodisiac. To be intimate, we need to feel appreciated and accepted for who we are.***

We often find it easier to practice kindness with our friends and our children then we do a long-term partner. We accept our friends for who they are, despite their mistakes and foibles, but for many couples, your partner seems like a walking pile of faults that need correcting. Let it go. If you are over 50, face it, your partner is not going to change in any substantial way. Try to see your partner's less than ideal traits as areas to be supported, understood and helped. When both you and your partner take this same approach, then your love life as well as the rest of your life will improve.

How do you do that? You could start by not saying stupid things. We are all growing older, and no one has abs like they used to, or the pointy breasts of a 20-year-old. No one, man or women, will appreciate being compared negatively to someone else, even if that someone is an earlier version of themselves. If you want to get naked with your partner then you are attracted to who they are today, so make sure they know how handsome or beautiful you find them.

Both men and women want to be appreciated. If they've done something nice, let them know how you feel about that. Make your partner know that you don't take for granted all that they do for you or your family. We all want to feel noticed and cherished.

Respect goes hand in hand with kindness. Show your partner that you respect who they are, even if their opinions and choices sometimes differ from yours. Make them feel valued, loved and cherished for who they are.

[**Michael**] *Guys, a simple formula to a women's heart is to pay attention. Know about her work, and her friends. Know her favorite flower. Remember that she takes her tea with two sugars and no milk. Notice when she's changed her hair or her clothes. You don't need a grand gesture; these little things may get you more traction than a trip to the Bahamas. Also, just listen. Listening without trying to "fix it," will get you a lot farther than, well, trying to "fix it." I know you have a solution to everything, but this is the time to keep your brilliance to yourself.*

Leave your partner a sexy note. Cook them their favorite food. Spend five minutes each day thinking of ways to make your partner happy. Remember this isn't transactional. If your attitude is "I'm being nice, so I expect you to have sex with me," then you aren't being kind, you're being manipulative. Understand your partner. Men and women have different psychologies. Women often need to feel loved and protected before they can feel intimate and sexual. Men often feel that sex is how they know their partner loves them. You're never going to change your partner's basic psychology, but understanding each other will lead to having a better love life. When partners are kind, considerate and respectful of each other, it is easy for them to feel valued and the biggest barrier to a wonderful love life will be removed.

[Michael] *Julia and I met on eHarmony. Isn't that modern? Something that mutually attracted us was that in our respective eHarmony profiles we each had a story about people in our lives who had the kind of marriages that we aspired to. In my case, I told about my Uncle Frank and Aunt Lydia, and how if you spent more than 10 minutes with my Uncle Frank, he was likely to say something nice about his wife, whether she was in the room or not. Conversely, if you spent more than 10 minutes with my Aunt Lydia, she was likely to say something nice about her husband, whether or not he was in the room.*

The moral here is to praise your mate to others. Be your partner's best cheerleader. When your partner hears from others the nice things you've said about them, that will give them the feeling of emotional comfort and safety that we all need to "Be Here Now."

HIS ERECTIONS

So ladies, how many things do we have to be self-conscious about? Our bellies? Our breasts? Or how about our thighs, buttocks, hair, eyebrows, and eyelashes? Let's not forget those random chin hairs that seem to sprout up overnight.

Yes we women have plenty of things to be sensitive about (even though we don't have to be—and don't need to be—see the "Confidence" section). But for a man, it's all about the penis. A man has more of his self-worth tied up in his penis than he does in his stomach, legs, wrinkly skin and balding head put together, and if for any reason his penis isn't working up to specifications, it can be like a boot to the testicles for him. Trust us on this: he is really sensitive about his penis.

You may remember your partner bragging about his length and girth, and his ability to save the day when he needed to change a tire and was missing a jack handle. You may remember when all you had to do was breath in his ear to watch it rise, and rise, and rise; taut and firm like it was ready to explode.

If your partner is over 50, it is virtually assured that things have changed, at least somewhat, and likely to change more in the years to come. You may find that his erection waxes and wanes during sex, that he has more trouble coming to climax. You may find that he has days where it won't rise at all.

All right, let's get the most important point over right at the start. **This is Not About You.** He is not waning because you are not desirable enough. He is not soft because you don't have quite the taut body you used to. He wanted to get naked with you; he wants you. He may want you so terribly he can taste it, but that won't make things rise if the blood flow isn't there.

> *His inability to get an erection is NOT because he doesn't find you desirable. It's not your fault, and it's not his fault. It's a plumbing issue.*

Erection problems are common to older men, which is why relieving that problem is a multi-billion dollar industry. You both need to understand the changes that you might expect, and understand that great sex and true passion do not require an ever-ready rock-hard penis. In any case, his inability is likely due to a big dinner, too much alcohol or a host of other common causes. See "How to Have an Erection After 50."

First, read and have him read "You Are Not Your Penis," and second, be kind. No matter how intellectually enlightened he is over what is a perfectly normal aging problem, he is going to be sensitive. If you are a little disappointed that the evening won't go as you had hoped, know that he is at least twice as disappointed.

[Michael] *Of course you want to help, and you may feel that massaging his limp penis or sucking it might help bring him to full erection. If he's nicely plump or half hard, that might be just the trick.*

But if he's really soft, it can be frustrating or embarrassing because it focuses on the problem, and makes him feel worse that nothing is happening.

When things are just not happening for him down there, it is best to switch the focus off of him completely. Let him work on his head technique, take an hour and find just that combination of tongue and breath and touch that sends your head spinning. Have him give you a full-body hot oil massage. You aren't being greedy, because making you happy is the best way to make him happy. Seriously. And don't be surprised if a little time between your legs or sitting on your naked rear massaging you won't be the solution to the problem he really wants to solve anyway.

YOU ARE NOT YOUR PENIS

[**Michael**] *Yes, yes, I know. There was a time when your erection would pop up unbidden at the mere sight or scent of a woman, or even while watching Mary Ann bake coconut cream pies on Gilligan's Island. In bed with the partner of your choice, you could sport a tent pole strong enough to hold the tarp shading a family of 12 at a picnic. When you ejaculated, you had to call for the second towel.*

And now things are different. Your penis seems to have joined a union when you weren't looking and occasionally now takes coffee breaks at inconvenient times. Sometimes he is as likely to rise out of bed as a teenager asked to take the trash out at 7 a.m. Forget the second towel, a single tissue can handle the mess now. Maybe half a tissue.

Do you feel this makes you less of a man? Do you fear your performance every time you slide under the covers? Well, let's put this in perspective. Do you wear reading glasses? Are you less of a man because the lens in your eye has stiffened with age and can't focus on the book you're reading? (Irony: lens too stiff, penis not stiff enough.) Do you sport gray hair on your temples, assuming you still have hair? Why weren't you enough of a man to keep your hair follicles from running out of hair dye? A real man would keep his hair follicles in line!

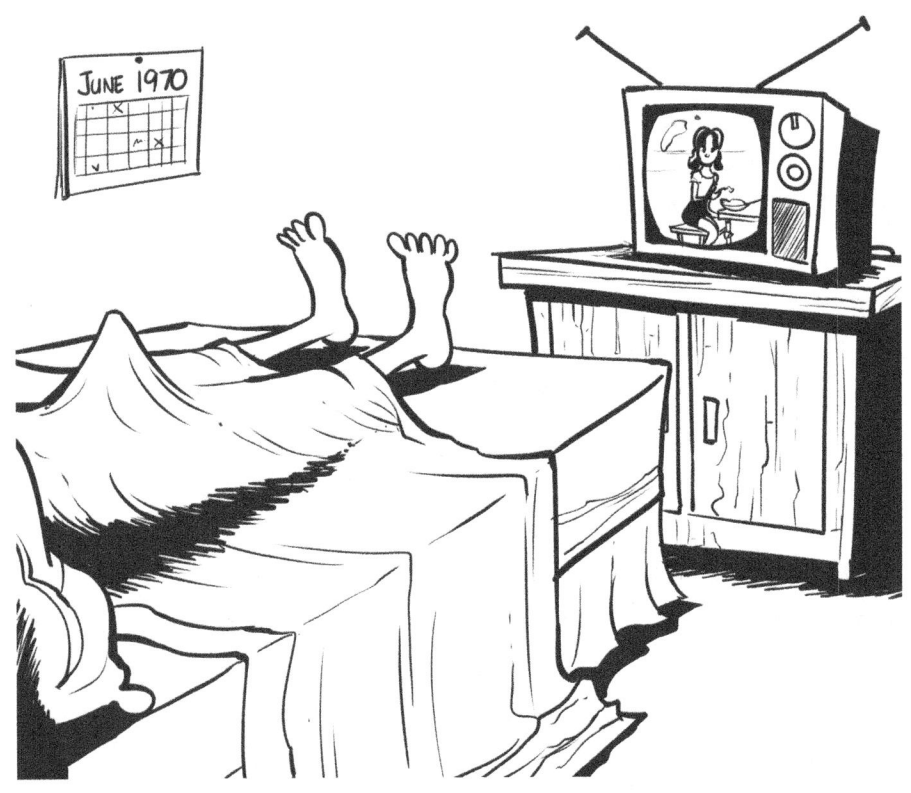

OK, so here are some truths. Your body is changing. Does this feel like fifth-grade health class now? All the guys your age are facing the same issues, and knowing you as the above-average guy that I do, you're better off than most. Not only that, but **you cannot control your erections.** *He doesn't go up when you want him to, he goes up when he's ready. For instance, on times when mine will just not work, despite best handling, my wife and I know that I may be getting a cold or virus that will show up a day or two later. You see, my body apparently*

prioritizes functions, and at the first sign of stress, it hoards its resources and throws out "unnecessary" services. I know that I'm not in charge of my erections, because if I was, I would re-prioritize bodily functions, and put erections just one notch below breathing.

Let it go. This is not your fault, and you're certainly no less of a man for surviving life long enough to deal with these changes. The good news is, you can still have smoking-hot sex. You can create an environment that will give your penis the care it needs to come out on its own. You can create the right attitude to deal with the occasional penis vacation day, and soon after you'll be crying, "Coach, let me back in the game." You can crawl into bed knowing that, whatever happens, you can have a great time. After all, an hour spent naked with your lover adds an hour to your life, regardless of what else happens.

*[**Julia**] When Michael and I are in bed together and it becomes clear that actual intercourse is not in the cards for him, we have some choices to make. We can either switch the focus to my pleasure (often incorporating a favorite sex toy), or we can decide to connect in other ways that don't require him to have an erection, whether that is just holding and kissing each other, giving or getting massages, or just cuddling up and talking. I never chalk these nights up to the "Failure" category. They are all "Wins" because we took the time to be together and were able to connect in some way.*

If we as women make our men feel we are disappointed if they can't perform, all we are going to do is add to their performance anxiety. This will be a self-fulfilling prophecy. The goal should always be connection, not climax. After all, how often does it happen that you fail to climax as part of your sexual experience? Do you feel like some sort of horrible failure as a result? I sure hope not. Do you want your partner to feel like a failure because he couldn't find the magic combination that night to send you to the proverbial moon? Of course not. Take the time to be with one another, regardless of how things play out. Take in the joy of your connection.

HOW TO HAVE AN ERECTION AFTER 50

[Michael] *To grow the regular erections you want, you need to learn some gardening skills. Decades ago, erections were like weeds, popping up overnight anywhere their seeds landed, without effort, water or care. Now, erections are more like hot-house tomatoes. No, that's not right. Cucumbers. I meant cucumbers. To grow a healthy specimen, you need to prepare the soil and give it the right amount of water, sun and fertilizer. Your cucumber may take a bit longer to grow to full size than your previous weedy efforts, but it will be more appreciated when it's ready for use. Put a prize ribbon on it and take it to the fair.*

Blood flow. Your cucumbers need water, your penis needs blood flow. Anything that effects blood flow may interfere with your fun. Exercise can increase blood flow. Some men find that regular exercise or even exercise right before sex may help keep the blood and juices flowing. Losing weight can help. You've been thinking about losing that extra poundage for years, what better reason could you have? Exercise and losing weight can increase blood flow, but a lot of common things will reduce it, including:

- *Eating a big meal. Think about saving dinner for after sex, or eat lightly.*
- *Lots of fatty, fried, and processed foods can decrease blood circulation throughout the body. A recent study showed that ED was uncommon among men who ate a traditional Mediterranean*

diet, one including fruits, vegetables, whole grains and healthy fats.[7] Eat right.

- *Smoking*
- *Too much alcohol. While a little may help loosen you up and put you "in the mood," too much will restrict your blood flow.*
- *High blood pressure*
- *Stress*
- *Not enough sleep*
- *Certain antidepressants, narcotic pain relievers, blood pressure medications, and antihistamines can cause problems with your erection. If this is the case, check with your doctor. Your doctor may be able to put you on a lower dose, or there may be another drug that works as well but doesn't have sexual side effects.*

Another thing you might need to change: Your attitude. You may not be able to control growing an erection, but you certainly have the ability to shrink one. Here is one tip you should put in all CAPS, underlined, bolded and in bright red: The best way to lose an erection is to worry that you are going to lose an erection.

The best way to lose an erection is to worry that you are going to lose an erection.

How do you adopt a more relaxed attitude? Let it go. Let it all go. Read "You are not your Penis" above. Go to bed with no expectations

---

[7] https://www.premiermedicalhv.com/news/mediterranean-diet-can-help-patients-erectile-dysfunction/

other than spending a little skin-to-skin time with your lover. How do you stop worrying and imagining those scenes of wilting asparagus? You need to get out of your head. Live the moment you are in, lose your self-consciousness, and feel the sensations of the moment. Read "Be Here Now" for tips on losing the spinning dialog in your head. A little legal cannabis may help to shut down that voice and increase sensation. Read "Sex and Cannabis."

Also, have patience. As you grow older, it is totally normal for things to take longer to get going, even when you are skin-to-skin. If things are starting slowly, I often find that going down on my wife does the trick, engaging my senses of taste and scent as well as touch. A little slippery sliding silicone lube can be nice, and check out our tip for keeping hot lube readily at hand. In addition, a much better scene in your mind than wilting asparagus is imagining the hot sex to come, or replaying some of your favorite memories. This is one of the many reasons to schedule times for sex. If you know that you've set aside the evening for fun, the anticipation will build in your mind, and you may notice a happy swelling as the appointed hour grows near.

However, even with the best sunlight and water, your garden may need some fertilizer. If so, go to a doctor, and find options that will work for you. Viagra, Cialis, and a host of variants have provided almost 1.7 billion orgasms since their introduction in 2002. OK, I just made that part up. But needless to say these drugs have provided more happiness to more people than cat pictures on the Internet and Steve Martin combined. Are you less of a man because you are taking advantage of these marvelous, magic remedies? Of course not. Your body is changing. Think of this as reading glasses for your penis, or perhaps more aptly, like a vibrator for your partner. And if you think it's a loss that your partner wants a little vibratory help to bring her to sweet orgasmic peak, then you haven't read the rest of this book. Her body is changing as well.

Finally, illness or injury can foil our best efforts. But that does not mean the end. As the previous chapter noted "You are Not Your Penis," you are a man and can still please your partner and enjoy many steamy and passionate times to come. In fact, when things aren't working at all, forget about yourself and focus on pleasing your lover. If you leave her sexually satisfied, she isn't going to consider today's lack of erection to be a big deal at all. Play the hand you've been dealt for all its worth, even if all you have is a pair of twos, you can still hit the jackpot.

AROUSAL AND LUBRICATION

Men and women are different. Maybe you've heard this? Both men and women need to be mentally aroused to have great sex or even to want to have sex at all. Mental arousal for a man, regardless of whether his penis is erect, comes on very quickly, perhaps measured in seconds from the time his lover drops her robe.

Mental arousal for women is usually a much slower process—and much easier to get off track. To begin with, a woman feels vulnerable in lovemaking, and unless she feels loved and safe, she is unlikely to feel aroused. (See our "Kindness" section.) Secondly, it is difficult for a woman to let go of the hundred things that need doing that were floating around her head before you began to take off any clothing. You'll find many helpful hints on how to stop the mental spinning in our "How to Be Here Now" section. But the key lesson here is that for great lovemaking, you need to take the time to allow a slow simmer to come to a rolling boil.

For great sex, you must have both arousal and lubrication. A woman who is post-menopausal may naturally lubricate less when aroused, and will have thinner vaginal walls that are more prone to damage. Therefore, to avoid pain during sex, or even to avoid injury, a woman needs sufficient lubrication. While a woman who is aroused will normally lubricate, this is not always true. The amount that a woman lubricates varies widely from woman to woman, and some women can be very mentally and physically aroused without having sufficient lubrication for sex. This is an important point, as some people link lubrication to arousal and assume that if they or their partner are not lubricating, they are not aroused, which is not necessarily the case.

Conversely, a woman who is producing lubrication is not necessarily aroused. The body is strange, and some women will lubricate without being aroused when they realize they are about to have intercourse, even at times in the extreme case of rape, perhaps as part of the body's defense mechanisms.

Regarding arousal, that is the focus of much of the rest of this book. Take your time. Start foreplay the day before. Read "How to Be Here Now," and "Building Anticipation – Mental Foreplay." Anything worth having is worth the effort to keep it. A wonderful sex life is one of the greatest gifts you can give each other. Put in the effort to make it happen.

Also, use the language that is going to entice your lover rather than turn them off. See the section on "What Do I Call It?" What do the words cunt, twat, pussy, cock, dick, and prick have in common? They are also words of abuse and derision. Find that special language of love that makes you both feel wanted and adored. It doesn't matter if other people would find his "manhood," or her "jade garden" to be silly terms. This is intimate and personal, you don't need to post it on Facebook.

Regarding lubrication, women who don't lubricate sufficiently once aroused will need artificial lube. The rest of us don't need it—we just want it! Smooth, slippery, sensual lubes are not only a necessity for some women but a great addition to sexual experience for all lovers.

See our section on "All About Lube," and find the product that is right for you.

Aside from slow, steamy foreplay, a woman can also help herself to become aroused and lubricate. "Use it or lose it" is a real thing when it comes to sexual health, and the more sex you have—including masturbation—the easier it will be to become aroused, and the better health your vagina will be in. Some women find they become aroused easier by exercising before sex, and a study from the University of Texas at Austin found that watching erotic films could bring on arousal. Of course most women don't need to read a study to know that reading something erotic or watching something sexy can start the juices flowing. For many women, this will mean something north of porn, which may feel degrading and humiliating to watch. Erotica involves more romance and mystery, as well as more respect and mutuality.

Even if a woman is fully aroused and lubricating, it is still possible for sex to be painful. Talk to your doctor, and if necessary a specialist in these specific issues. There is a whole sub-specialty of physical therapy focused exclusively on pelvic pain. If this is a problem for you, you are definitely not alone. But most importantly, don't give up! There are plenty of ways to end up spent in total sexual satisfaction without intercourse. Experiment, read our section on "Mating Rituals," and adapt as needed. If you come up with a great ritual, write us and maybe we'll put it in the revised edition of this book.

[Michael] *A last word to the guys on lubrication and pain during sex. If you want to be a great lover, DO NOT use porn as a guide. Porn is mostly made for guys, and a strong window-shaking pounding looks* *better visually than slow, hot, and steamy sex. Do you think your partner loves it when you jackhammer her hard? Think again. Women may put up with it because they think you want it, but most women prefer it slow, smooth and luscious. If she wants a stronger pounding, she'll let you know, but a post-menopausal woman has thinner vaginal walls and is slower to lubricate, so she could get hurt in the process. If you are looking for a better sex life, a trip to the emergency room is most definitely not the way to start. Do her a favor, unplug the jackhammer.*

ALL ABOUT LUBE

As we spoke of in the section on "Her Lubrication," any woman past menopause is likely to take longer and require more foreplay to lubricate, and her body will provide less lubrication when she does. Luckily, the days of Johnson's baby oil and whipping cream have given way to a wide selection of products of every texture and flavor designed to enhance your lovemaking. In this section, we will look at the three major categories of lubes: water-based, oil-based and silicone-based, and outline the pluses and minuses of each.

Something we won't cover but should let you know about is that women suffering vaginal pain may get relief from doctor-prescribed lubes with analgesic compounds. We will also look at the many ways that lube can enhance your lovemaking other than just replacing or augmenting natural vaginal lubrication. And some of the ways you can use lube may surprise you. We love this stuff. We buy quart-sized bottles of Pjur Light Bodyglide silicone lube and refill our smaller bottles as needed. Visit www.cheaplubes.com to see a selection that will have your head spinning. And don't worry—the boxes come with a very discreet return address so no one will be the wiser!

Water-based lubes: Water-based lubes are water soluble and widely available. Think of the classic K-Y Jelly. Water-based lubes generally include either glycerin, which results in a sort of sweet taste, or parabens or propylene glycol. Water-based lubes with synthetic glycerin have been known to trigger yeast infections in women who are prone to them. Water-based lubes containing parabens or propylene glycol can irritate sensitive skin, and without the sweet glycerin may have a somewhat bitter taste.

The Pros of Water-based Lubes: They are easy to find, inexpensive, safe to use with latex condoms and, unless specifically colored, will not stain fabric. Being water-soluble, they are easy to clean off your body and sheets. Water-based lubes are compatible with all sex toys, wash off toys easily, and come in a wide variety of flavors, including chocolate.

The Cons of Water-based Lubes: The water part of the lube will evaporate pretty quickly, and often leaves a sticky or tacky surface that is definitely not sexy. How fast this happens depends on the humidity. While it might last through your full sex experience in New Orleans, here in the dry Rocky Mountains where we live we find that water-based lubes can get sticky in a matter of minutes. You can re-wet the lube by adding water or saliva, but of course that can interrupt the flow of the sexual experience. (Although it might also enhance it if done strategically!) Since it is water soluble, it's not a great choice for the bath tub, shower or hot tub, as the slipperiness is easily washed off.

Silicone-based lubes: This is our favorite. Silicone-based lubes last the longest of all and are especially recommended for women with chronic vaginal dryness or genital pain. Silicone lubes are generally considered hypo-allergenic, and are not absorbed by the skin or mucous membranes. Most silicone-based lubricants are certified latex-condom safe, and this is the type of lube used in pre-lubricated condoms. Silicone lube is mostly found online or at your local sex shop, rather than in your local drug store.

The Pros of Silicone-based Lubes: They have a lovely silky feeling. They last a long time. Since it is not water soluble, it's a great solution for water play, hot tubs, showers and warm oceans. It is not absorbed by the skin or mucous membranes.

The Cons of Silicone-based Lubes: They can damage silicone-based sex toys, since frequent use could damage the surface, making it sticky or gummy to the touch, or stretching the surface out over time so that it is no longer holding the original shape. When vibrators get slack, it is harder to feel the vibration. Many silicone sex toys will have warnings regarding use with silicone lubes. We have actually found this to be a fairly minor problem, if you wash sex toys immediately after use—as you should. While better than oil-based lubes, silicone lube can stain fabric, and compared to water or oil-based lubes it is more expensive. If you want to do that full-body baby oil experience that used to take a full $5 bottle of Johnson's & Johnson's, that same experience with silicone lube could set you back $50. Being non-water soluble has its downsides, as it takes a good shower with soap to get it off. We recommend covering your sheets with a soft fleece blanket to protect them during play time.

Oil-based lubes: Oil-based lubes may be natural and even found in your kitchen, such as olive, almond or coconut oil, or they may be synthetic or petroleum based, such as mineral oil, Vaseline, and body lotions.

The Pros of Oil-based Lubes: These are inexpensive and easy to find. Natural oil-based lubes are safe for skin or mucous membranes. If you can put it in your mouth, it's probably safe for your labia.

The Cons of Oil-based Lubes: These are not safe for latex condoms, as they make the latex porous and prone to ripping or breaking. Synthetic or petroleum-based lubes can irritate the vulva, stain fabric and are hard to clean.

OK, now that you've chosen your favorite lube to help with a lack of natural lubrication during vaginal intercourse, let's talk about other really fun ways to use lube.

- Use it when you masturbate by hand. Just a few drops can turn a rough hand job into silky, wet smoothness.

- Use is when you masturbate with a vibrator. You'll find that the fluid, gently gliding sensation is a total game-changer.

- Use a few drops inside a condom. If you put a drop or two inside the condom before you unroll it, you can unlock a world of sensual feeling for the man, and it should be enough to shut him up about how the condom "ruins sex" for him. Just be careful not to overdo this as you don't want to risk having the condom slip right off during sex.

- Use lots of it during anal sex. It is hopefully obvious, but there is no natural lubrication at all during anal sex, and while you might find you can put on too much lube during vaginal sex (Help—he keeps slipping out!), when it comes to the rear end, too much is never enough.

- Use it during fellatio. This may sound counterintuitive, but sometimes it's hard for a woman to muster up enough spit to provide sufficient wetness. A flavored lube can provide a different experience for her and may keep her jaw from getting as tired. This is one place where a nicely flavored water-based lube could work really well.

- Use it during cunnilingus. What's good for the gander is good for the goose. As a general rule, the slipperier the better and sometimes the tongue is just not wet enough.

- Use it everywhere. Sexy massages, touching anywhere and everywhere. There are few better sensations than two steamy, slippery bodies writhing together in a white-hot heat. We sometime visualize a giant sexual slip-n-slide when gliding against each other. Now that is some serious grown-up fun! See our tip on how to have hot oil at-the-ready under the "Ready and Waiting" section. And if you haven't experienced the sexual heat and anticipation of having hot oil dripped drop by drop onto your skin, well, you should. Maybe keep some inexpensive sheets or lay down a thick washable fleece blanket for your all-out oil fests. Find a great lube that works for you, get yourself a frequent buyer's card and keep stocked up! You'll thank us later.

Final word – Clitoral arousing gels. These are products meant to increase blood flow to your genitals, making it easier to orgasm. They often have ingredients such as menthol, peppermint, or almond oil. They don't really work for us, but many women swear (and swear loudly) by them. From what we understand, like cannabis, more is not always better. A tiny drop may be wonderful, but too much can have you crawling out of your skin and hurriedly finding a wet washcloth. Women who are sensitive to fragrances will want to avoid the menthol and peppermint varieties for sure.

SEX TOYS AND ORGASMS

[Julia] *I remember going to my friend Michelle's house one day when I was about 11 years old. She had recently discovered a little contraption in her parents' bedroom and wanted to show it to me. It had two little straps that fit over your hand and a power button. When activated, the little machine started to vibrate. We took turns putting it against different parts of our bodies, somehow intuiting that this was meant to provide some sort of massage. I tried it against my arm, the tops of my legs, my belly, and then, randomly, on my crotch. HooHee! We have a winner!*

It would be several years before I felt the pleasure of that first orgasm again, but it certainly left an impression. Ironically, though my first orgasm was produced through the use of a vibrator, I spent the next several decades ignoring the benefits or uses of sex toys. To me they seemed somehow dirty—something naughty women used—and also like a copout or insult to the skills of my lovers.

It wasn't until I was well into my 40s (or maybe even my early 50s?) that I decided to see what all the fuss was about. Michael convinced me that it might be a fun thing to add to the mix for us.

As we age, it definitely takes more work to build up enough sexual energy to have a satisfying orgasmic release. I found myself feeling guilty during sex that things were taking me so long. And as soon as you start to worry that your fun is becoming a chore for your partner, you are out of the moment, into your head, and almost certain to lose the excitement you were in the process of building.

This is where the vibrator comes in, or what I have come to affectionately call "The Closer." Now I can enjoy all the sexy buildup I want with my partner but when we feel like we are ready to take things to their natural conclusion, we bring in our little electronic reinforcement.

We have learned to build the vibrator in to our sex play in a way that feels natural and mutual. We continue to stay connected (whether literally by still having intercourse but with the vibrator strategically placed between us and against my clitoris, or figuratively if we are focusing more on me at the moment but my lover is the one gently positioning the vibrator to the place of maximum pleasure for me). It is in no way a copout on our sexual prowess. Quite the contrary, we have learned to incorporate it to magnify our pleasure. And in the end, what my lover wants for me is some mind-bending squeals of delight. He doesn't really care whether those squeals were produced with or without battery-powered assistance.

On a scale of one to ten for where I would place vibrators in my sexual fun toolbox, I give it an 11. As my eyes started to age I added reading glasses. If someone's hearing has faded, they would use hearing aids. There is no reason to feel any differently about using a vibrator.

You might feel intimidated by the wide array of shapes, sizes, colors and functions available on the market today. This is completely understandable. It is intimidating. But don't let that stop you from taking advantage of this incredibly versatile tool. It is worth the trip outside your comfort zone. Read on for how to get over the hump and on your way to orgasmic bliss.

[Michael] *Would you like to have more sex? Give your partner what she needs, wake up her body, and she'll come back for more and more. There are no rules about how to help a woman climax. If intercourse alone brings her to orgasm, great, but only a minority of women can orgasm with intercourse alone, and that minority gets smaller as we age. If masturbating her with your oiled fingers brings on the climax, wonderful. If sucking her clitoris and running your tongue through her labia while massaging her g-spot causes those screams of joy, fantastic.*

As a woman ages, it's very common for her to take longer to orgasm. No matter how great a lover you are, if it takes too long she'll begin to worry about you. "I'm embarrassed this is taking so long," she might think. "Is this a chore for him? What is he thinking?," Once she becomes self-conscious, and can't "Be Here Now," the pleasure part of her evening is over.

Don't let her lose the moment. A great vibrator, especially a couple's vibrator or vibrating cock ring where you are both fully engaged, isn't a replacement for you, it's an enhancement, a super power. Don't start the evening right off with a sex toy as she can get "buzzed out" if you start too early. But once the juices are fully flowing, and she's panting in your ear, activate your super power and remind her what total satisfaction feels like. Taking your hearing aids out at this point may be a smart move. Safety first.

LET'S VISIT A SEX STORE

If your idea of an adult toy store is some dank space in the sleazy part of town with sticky floors where people go to anonymously rent porn, think again. In many towns, ours included, stores that cater to sexual accoutrements are in mainstream strip malls with brightly lit tasteful and colorful displays, knowledgeable and candid sales people, and customers you might otherwise bump into on your stop in to the local Whole Foods.

You could certainly explore your options on-line and buy something that way, but we highly encourage you to make the trip to a local store if you have that option in your area. Being able to pick up and touch the various options will go a long way toward helping you guess at the kind of toy you might enjoy the most.

And those young, hip, overly pierced salespeople are so comfortable with their own sexuality that you will forget about your own queasiness. They know their stuff, and have no compunction about talking openly and honestly about the wares they sell.

First, go to the right store. A great sex store will be clean and brightly lit and have a large selection of vibrators from reputable brands like We-Vibe, Lelo, Jimmy Jane, and Je Joue, and great lubes from companies like Pjur and ID. Don't be freaked out at a few whips and leather corsets, as all stores need to cater to a wide variety of customer tastes. You want to be able to handle the vibrator and check out the feel and vibrations, so find a store that provides test units to play with. Also, do they know their stuff? A great sex store will have female sales people who know their products, ahem... intimately. Ask questions, and don't be embarrassed.

Our local store told us that more than 20 percent of their clientele was over 60, and that's in a major college town. Believe us, they've heard it all. A good salesperson will be able to give you honest, detailed advice and be unashamed and enthusiastic about helping you find what will work best for you.

Second, don't buy a cheap vibrator! A good vibrator will probably cost a $100 or more. Government regulation has yet to come to the sex toy industry, and materials that would not be allowed in children's toys such as phthalates and mercury can sometimes be found in cheap vibrators. Avoid any toys that have a strong chemical smell, or are marked "for novelty use only." The phrase "for novelty use only" allows the manufacturer to avoid what little regulation exists in this area by pretending that it will never actually be used in or on the body. Avoid anything with sticky, jelly rubber and stick to medical-grade silicone, which is non-porous and easy to clean with soap and water, or perhaps hard plastic from a reputable brand. You are putting this in literally the most sensitive place in your body. Aren't you worth it?

Third, pick the one that is right for you. The first thing is aesthetics. Buy something that gives you a sexy tingle to look at, not some scary, garish device with ridges and knobs more suited to anal probing by Aliens. Go for sleek and sensual. Will you use it in the bath tub, hot tub or shower? If so, you'll want a vibrator that is waterproof. Is it too noisy? If you still have kids or other non-dog persons at home, a loud vibrator may make you lose your "Be Here Now" vibe as you worry about whether the sound is carrying through the house. Multiple vibratory modes allow you to find the setting that's right for you. Another important feature is battery life, especially as we often take longer to orgasm as we age. Having a vibrator suddenly conk out just as you are rising to a dramatic peak is *really* frustrating, and we speak from experience here.

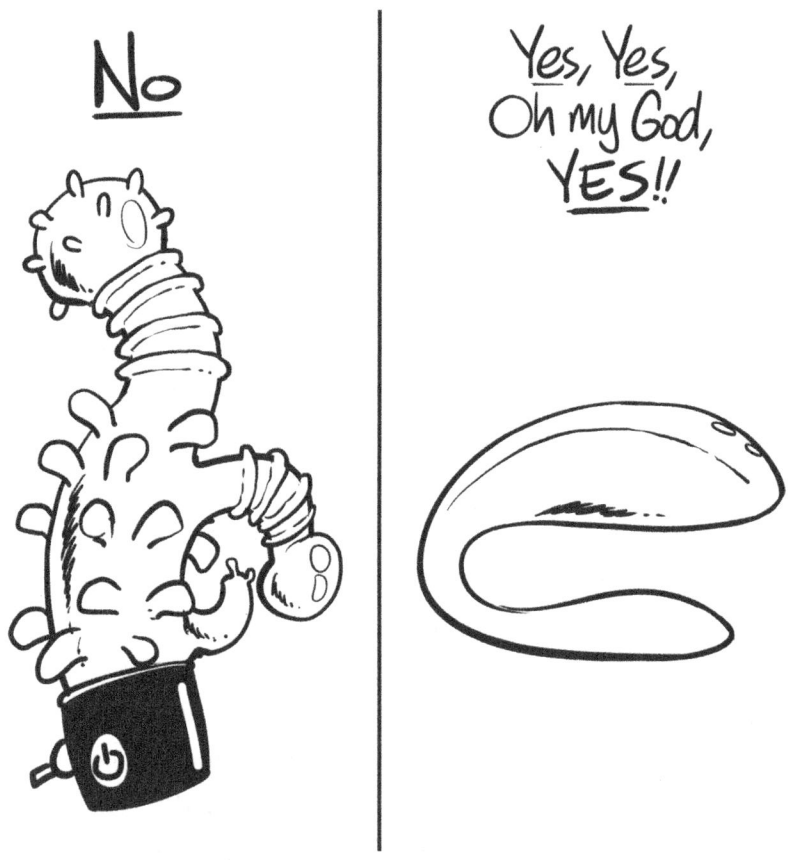

How do you want to use it? If you are flying solo for the time being, then you may want an insertable vibrator or dildo to get the feeling of penetration. If it has been some time since you've had sex your vagina may have atrophied, so be careful of size. Seventy percent of all women need clitoral stimulation to orgasm, and "rabbits" are vibrators designed to simultaneously provide penetration as well as clitoral stimulation. Many women flying solo find that small sleek vibrators and bullets meant specifically for clitoral and vulvar stimulation work wonderfully well, and are also quite discreet. In fact, some bullet vibrators are made specifically to mimic tubes of lipstick.

Some vibrators are specifically made for couple's play. The We-Vibe sync, for example, has a sort of 'U' shape, with one end going inside the vagina along with your partner's penis (if you like), while the other end stays external to massage your clitoris. We often just sort of mash it between us atop Julia's clitoris while we are coupled, skipping the insertion option.

Another good option is a vibrating cock ring. While the word "cock" may turn you off and make you feel like this is too hard-core, it is actually a very elegant solution with an overly crass name. Cock rings are ring-shaped vibrators designed to slip over the man's penis, resting at the base of the shaft. A small vibrator sits at the top of this ring so that when the man's penis is inside his lover's vagina, the vibrator is perfectly positioned to provide clitoral stimulation. In addition, the vibration action ends up making the whole penis vibrate to a degree, so you are getting some seriously good vibrations inside and out. Cock rings also have the advantage of not slipping off your oiled body at an inconvenient time, and the compression ring around your partner's penis (or penis and testicles, depending on the model) may help to keep your partner erect longer.

We recommend avoiding the giant penis-substitute dildos altogether, as not only are these generally cheap and suspect toys, but also your partner may not appreciate being compared to a porn star's probably artificially enlarged replica erection. You also want to make sure you have the right intensity level, as some vibrators just don't have the "oomph" you need. Test the vibrator in the store on your hand, or even against the more sensitive tip of your nose.

There is another class of sex toy for women that may be worth looking into. Instead of vibration, this type of toy uses a gentle suction motion to stimulate the clitoris. It is supposed to mimic the feeling of oral sex. A very popular version of this has the most unfortunate name: "The Womanizer." Don't let the name scare you off, however. This baby has been called "the crack cocaine of sex toys." It is a great toy to use when you are alone, but it can also be incorporated into couple's sex play as well. In fact it is considered so effective that there is a prescription-only version approved by the FDA to treat low sexual desire and arousal issues.

If you have a partner, make toy shopping a date! The shopping itself becomes a naughty bit of foreplay, and you'll find yourself getting excited about trying out your new toy as you drive home together with your little classy gift bag sitting beside you.

WHAT ABOUT WHEN IT DOESN'T HAPPEN

So, you have set aside the night for play. You've warmed and darkened the room, started the music, lube and toys at the ready, and you've been looking forward to this all day—or even all week—and it just doesn't happen. Either one or both of you lack the energy or are so distracted you just can't get to the "Be Here Now" state.

First, make sure you've given it a real try, and that you've set the stage and "turned on the ons and off the offs" as suggested in our "Be Here Now" chapter. If it's the man who wants to quit because he can't get an erection but the woman is ready to go, then you can still give her a night to remember. See "How to Have an Erection after 50." Likewise, if the man is raring to go but the woman just can't quite get herself there, she may at least be game to snuggle up next to him while he (or she) masturbates him to a climax. Even if all you end up doing is cuddling and talking, chalk this up to a night of naked fun and connection. They won't all be home runs, but at least you showed up to play.

And don't give up too soon. There have been countless times that one or both of us has thought it wasn't going to happen, and after a slow, luscious massage and perhaps a toke or two of pot, we find to our surprise that we weren't quite as tired as we thought we were.

However, if it really doesn't work, don't worry. You get points for just showing up. This is no time to play the blame game. Even if you've been looking forward to this time, making a big deal out of it will only make your partner defensive and apprehensive for the next time. Just make a raincheck and set a future date for the next event, and turn the evening into something else that's fun and relaxing. Curl up on the couch, head in his lap, and watch an old black and white movie. Just have a little pot and have a giggle over good times past. Make a special dessert together. Take a bubble bath together.

MASTURBATION

It is a crime that so many of us think of masturbation as something dirty. Self-love is a joy that can stay with you your entire life. It's good for your health, good for your mood, and good for your love life. Unfortunately it is, at least in some circles, a term of abuse or derision. The British say "Wanker," another term for someone masturbating, when they mean "Idiot." See "What Do I Call It?" for the psychological damage caused by poor naming. We need a different language to describe what is a good, wholesome, healthful and joyous thing. We'll use the term "self-love" from here on out, but we would love to find a better term. Let us know if you have any suggestions.

> **"Having sex is like bridge. If you don't have a good partner, you'd better have a good hand." – Mae West.**

Self-love is real sex, and a vital skill—especially for women—as we age. It is a sad truth that as we get older there are less men than women, and not everyone can find a partner of their choice. By the time women are 75 or older, there are barely two men for every three women. Not only will self-love reduce pain and improve your mood, but think of it as sex insurance, keeping everything supple and operating in case you do meet a partner you want to share yourself with.

Sex, including self-love, involves gentle, range-of-motion exercises, which minimize pain and inflammation. Sex strengthens muscles around the joints, and helps to support them. Sex also releases endorphins, the body's natural pain relievers, and is naturally mood-elevating. What pill does all that?

And, you don't have to quit self-love if you have a partner. Self-love will help you understand your own body, understand what works and doesn't work for you. How can you expect your partner to find your pleasure buttons if you can't? Also, learning to masturbate your partner is a great skill to have. Some nights you may be just too tired for a full round of intercourse, but not too tired to enjoy a good hand job before drifting off to sleep with your lover. Learn about yourself, so that you can help him help you.

Most of the strategies we suggest in "How to Be Here Now," including the judicious use of legal pot, will help you make self-love a beautiful, sensual experience more likely to lead to total release. Thank God for "Grace and Frankie," the Emmy-nominated Netflix show starring Jane Fonda and Lily Tomlin, whose characters start a vibrator company specifically for older women, bringing to light the truth that not only do older people want and have sex, but that self-love is a beautiful thing limited only, in their case, by sex toys not designed for arthritic hands and poor eyesight.

The issue Jane Fonda and Lily Tomlin face on "Grace and Frankie" is a real one. Rheumatoid arthritis is three times as likely to happen to women as men. Look at vibrators from a cost-benefit perspective. If you can climax just by touching yourself and fantasizing, wonderful, but if it takes so long that pain from your aching joints takes you out of the moment, consider a vibrator.

Of course, artificial lubrication can help, as will fantasy. Fantasy isn't hurting you or your partner. No one needs to know what is happening inside of your head with one caveat: if you have a committed partner don't fantasize about people you know. It may be easy and tempting to fantasize about the woman up the street or that guy at the gym, but consciously fantasizing about someone you know will set your subconscious working to make it come true, and you may find yourself flirting with the object of your fantasy to the detriment of your relationship. Fantasizing about unavailable actors or musicians like George Clooney or Scarlet Johansson is unlikely to get you into trouble, unless you run in very different circles than we do. (Or unless like Ross on *Friends*, you actually happen to bump into Isabella Rossellini at the coffee shop.)

So, turn the lights down, turn the music up, take a warm bath and start to fantasize. Your happiness is literally in your own hands.

SENIOR VD – YES, YOU STILL NEED CONDOMS

If you are 55 or older, you were probably having your first sexual experiences before the HIV epidemic hit. VD was something sailors got traveling from port to port, and our worst fear was having to get shots for "The Clap." Many of us thought about condoms primarily as a way to avoid pregnancy.

Not anymore. As our kids and grandkids could tell us having been brought up on a continuing stream of information on safe sex, some venereal diseases are for life, and some can kill you. Venereal Disease is on the rise in the senior community, sometimes dramatically. It is almost as prevalent among people in their 60s as it is among people in their 20s. While more 20-somethings are sexually active, more are also using condoms. Us older folks, in contrast, are not. According to an Indiana study condom use among sexually active seniors over 60 is lower than any other age group.[8] Not only that, but as we get older our immune systems become weaker and have a harder time fighting off any disease or infection, and so avoiding infection becomes even more important as we age.

If you are single and sexually active, then don't just read this section but bone up on the mountain of information available online and in almost any medical clinic. The kids may find it hilarious to hear that Grandpa caught VD, but it isn't hilarious at all. Stay safe. Here are some tips to help you do so:

---

[8] http://www.nationalsexstudy.indiana.edu/

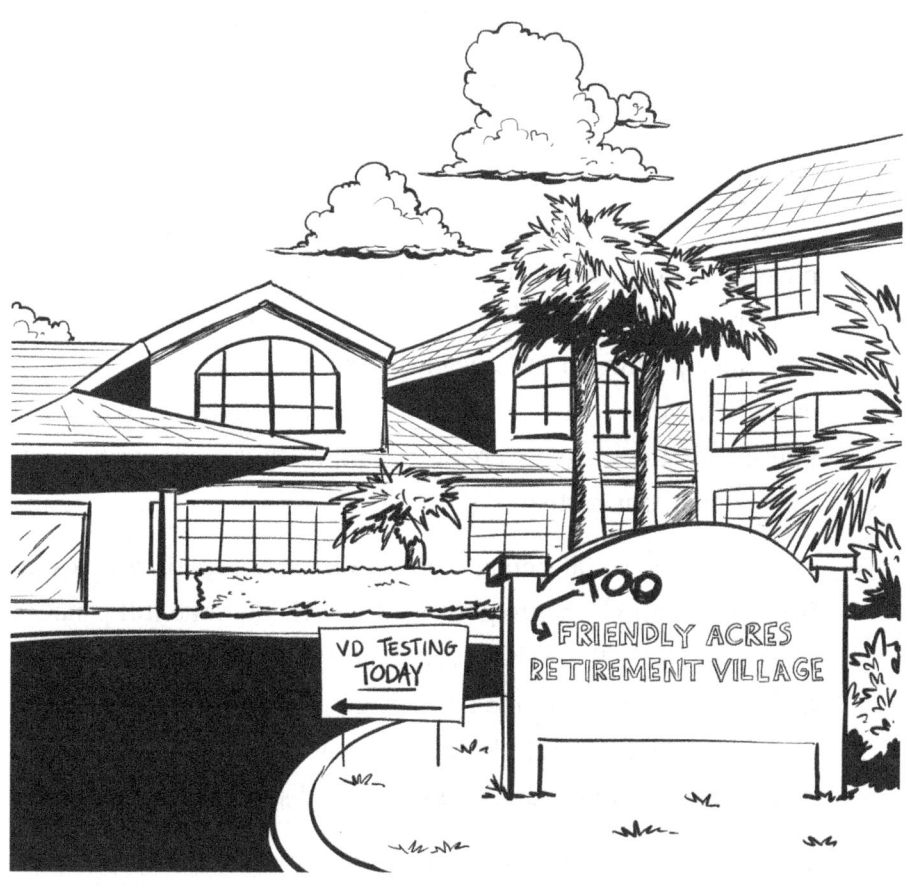

- Have the talk about condoms and VD before you take your clothes off. Even without teenage hormones fueling your sexual energy, we can still get "lost in the moment," and it only takes a moment to get infected. Also, have the talk while you have a clear head, not after your third martini or after a few tokes on that legal pot.

- Keep condoms with you if you are sexually active. Don't use the excuse of "we'll be fine just this once." Be prepared.

- Many STDs can be transmitted during oral or anal sex as well. Don't assume that if it's not vaginal sex that you have nothing to worry about. You should use dental dams (little latex rectangles you place over your partner's anus or vulva when giving oral pleasure) to protect yourself from such things as herpes, gonorrhea, syphilis and hepatitis if you are not in a monogamous relationship with an uninfected partner. If necessary, you can even DIY this—using a condom, rubber gloves or even non-porous plastic wrap to create a similar barrier between your tongue and your partner.

- Unless you are 100 percent sure you know a partner's sexual history, ask him or her to get tested for HIV and the full panel of STD's and have them show you the clean test results. If you are active with more than one partner, get yourself tested regularly. Luckily, since 2012, Medicare has provided for annual screenings for chlamydia, gonorrhea, and syphilis for free.

- If you have an STD, you must, must, must tell any potential partner before the clothes come off. If you care for them enough to have sex with them, you should care enough to be honest.

WHEN IT'S BEEN A LOOOONG TIME

If you picked this book up thinking "Incendiary Sex? Huh? You have got to be kidding. What about any sex at all?," you are far from alone. Most of the sections in this book, "How to Be Here Now," "Mating Rituals," and "Sex and Cannabis" are meant to take you from infrequent, boring and awkward sex to incendiary sex so passionate it will blow your mind. However, to begin that journey the starting point is that you both must be willing to get naked and try to have sex together, and many, many, couples just aren't there yet.

Maybe sex has just stopped between you two due to boredom, stress, changing bodies and sex drives, pain, or illness. Perhaps it's the fear of whether your partner is still turned on by you, or whether you can perform. Maybe the subject is so emotionally loaded that you fear saying *anything* that might cause the Elephant in the Room to go lumbering through the house, knocking over the furniture.

We can help. Some of that help is in other sections of this book. In the "Health" section we address illnesses and health problems that affect pain during sex and the libido. If the issue is fear of not getting an erection, read "His Erections," "You Are Not Your Penis," and "How to Have an Erection After 50" along with the "Health" section. If the fear is of painful or uncomfortable sex, read "Arousal and Lubrication," and "All About Lube."

In this section, we will give you tips on how to have that hard conversation, and help you shove the Elephant in the Room right out the door. We will show you how to get in touch with your own body, how the two of you can get in touch with each other, and also how a little legal pot may smooth the way for you both.

You want a better love life for you and your partner, right? Imagine how it could be. Isn't that worth a few uncomfortable conversations? Be bold (read our section on "Confidence"), be kind (read our section on "Kindness"), take a few notes here, and start down the road to a better life.

BREAKING THE ICE – HOW TO START THE CONVERSATION

There is probably no subject more loaded with emotional baggage than sex. More than kids, money, jobs and health. It cuts right to the most vulnerable core of us, to our sense of self and our deepest needs and insecurities. Sex is often at the core of the biggest, longest-lasting tensions in a relationship. These can last for decades, sucking the life out of an otherwise good relationship.

Talking about it should be a piece of cake, right? No, it probably won't be. But with love and a few strategies we will show you, you can clear the Elephant out of the room, with the result being a happier, more joyful, and more satisfying relationship. Isn't that worth some effort? If you could fix the happiness in your relationship with money, how much would you pay? Isn't your and your partner's happiness worth the time it takes to study the problem and find a solution?

Your happiness is important, so don't just do this off the cuff. Here are some suggestions and important Dos and Don'ts for having a difficult conversation about sex.

Suggestions

- You could start by announcing the conversation you'd like to have, "I'd like to talk to you about my feelings about sex," or " I know you care about me and want me to feel good, and I want to learn how to make you happy with sex, too, so I want to talk about how we can make it better. Is that OK with you?"

- You could also acknowledge that the topic may be sensitive or touchy, and that you may have different perspectives, but that you want to work together so you better understand one another.

- Other openings might include: "I've been thinking about ...," "What do you think about ...," "I want to have a better understanding of your thoughts about ..."

- You could write down your thoughts, and also your suggested solutions. You could ask your partner to read your words, and then you could discuss them.

- You could try having the discussion during a pleasant, private walk.

- If things get heated, it's better to stop and think about how to approach this better another time than to continue what might turn into a bad argument.

- Try to keep the focus on your love and connection. You want to keep the conversation about the positives, not the negatives. Contrast, "We never have sex anymore and I don't think I can live like this any longer" with something like, "Honey, I miss the closeness we used to feel and would love to find a way to get some of that back. Are you open to discussing this with me so we can come up with some possible solutions?"

While this book is about jump-starting your sex life, keep in mind that sex is something that may take a long time to build back up to. In fact, as ironic as it may seem, finding your way back to a regular sex life might require initially taking sex off the table completely. This will be the case if the thought of having sex again is triggering for you or your partner due to whatever baggage may be associated with it after all this time.

For these couples, the first step will be finding safe and non-threatening ways to slowly rebuild their physical and emotional connection. This will involve things like demonstrating kindness and respect for your partner, and finding ways to connect physically that do not involve actual sex. Hold hands. Go dancing. Exercise together. Or try your hand at many of the games we discuss below in the Mating Rituals section, but with some very firm ground rules. For example, you could try the breathing exercises (Tantra for Fun) or give each other sensual massages but do them with your clothes on if that makes you feel safer at first. Or experiment with putting a silky sheet between you and your partner so that actual sex is physically impossible, but you can still explore a little fun foreplay with one another. If you both agree "We will not have sex tonight," this could allow you each to feel freer in expressing yourselves romantically without worrying that by doing so you will be leading your partner on. If sex is off the table, you can give your lover that long passionate goodnight kiss and not fear that you are sending a mixed signal.

We make some suggested adjustments for couples trying to build their way back to intimacy in many of the games and exercises we describe below. The key is finding a way to make both of you feel safe in your attempt to explore and connect. Set the ground rules and be sure to stick to them so that your trust can grow. You can (and should) tweak the rules as your bond improves. Before you know it—you will be nuzzling up next to one another's naked bodies doing what nature intended all along.

The Dos

- DO be optimistic and positive, and expect the best from your partner. If you expect the discussion to go badly, it will.
- DO listen to your partner's ideas and opinions and consider them. Don't just be waiting for them to finish so you can talk.
- DO show respect for your partner. Don't talk down to them, and don't interrupt while they are speaking. Read our "Kindness" section.
- DO stop yourself from being defensive. Take a deep breath and come back with optimism and kindness. Watch your body language and unfold your arms.
- DO pick a neutral place to have a discussion. Not in a public place and certainly not in bed.
- DO turn off the electronics so you aren't interrupted or distracted.
- DO start sentences with "I," not "You."
- DO restate what you heard from your partner, to let them know you are listening, and to confirm that both of you understand what your partner is trying to say. "What I'm hearing you say is ___, is that accurate?"

- DO share memories of good times in the past. Try to remember some of your greatest sexual times together, like those steamy nights on your honeymoon.

- DO bring solutions. You may not end up with agreement on these, but it's important not just to talk about what's wrong, but to offer ideas on how to improve it. You will find many solutions in this book!

- DO try to come up together with a resolution and action plan.

- DO keep the conversation going. Your issues didn't happen in a day, and likely won't be solved in a day. Keep positive and keep talking over the coming weeks and months.

- If all of this feels too scary to you, it is OK to try to express your feelings in writing first. Frame it as a love letter to your partner in which you express your appreciation for all that you have and your desire to continue to grow together. Stay positive but get your message across that you feel the two of you could increase your love and satisfaction by putting some new emphasis on your physical and emotional connection.

The Don'ts

- DON'T trap your partner, as in having the conversation on a plane or car ride, or in a public place, unless that's what you both agreed to do. (We don't recommend this.)

- DON'T manipulate your partner. For instance, don't take your partner out to a nice dinner with the secret plan of having "the talk."

- DON'T ambush your partner as soon as they step in the door, or try an important conversation when there isn't enough time for a long conversation, or when your partner is tired or stressed.

- DON'T have a difficult conversation before or after sex.

- DON'T expect to have the talk immediately. If your partner wants some time to think about a topic, give it to them, but set a time and place that you will resume your talk within the next day or two.

- DON'T raise your voice or speak in anger.

- DON'T shame, blame, or complain. DON'T berate or belittle. DON'T come across as whiney or selfish. DON'T use sarcasm. DO go and read the "Kindness" section again. Got it?

- DON'T say "We Have to Talk," as it immediately brings up the hackles. "We have to talk about our horrible sex life" is a complete loser.

- DON'T say "you never" or "you always." These absolutes are maddening, especially to men, who can instantly think of at least one time that wasn't true, and fixate on that.

- DON'T add another discussion on top by doing a "and while we're at it…" If you wish your partner would pick up more around the house, pick another day to have that talk. One thing at a time.

Remember, you are worth it; your partner is worth it. Imagine how things could be. Show the elephant the door.

GETTING IN TOUCH WITH YOURSELF

Do you feel "broken"? Are you ashamed of your body, or worried your partner won't be turned on by you? Do you feel totally unsexual?

None of this is unusual, particularly for post-menopausal women. The hormones that were driving you to fill your womb and procreate, for which the sex was just a fun by-product, are fading or gone. Your body is changing, and none of us are what we were 30 or 40 years ago. What used to work just doesn't anymore.

However, the good news is that with new strategies all that can be turned around, and the first step is to love yourself. Let's begin by clearing up a few common misconceptions.

If you are a woman and were used to seeing your partner "rise to the occasion" at the drop of your robe, you may feel that his lack of instantaneous erection is a sign that he doesn't want you anymore. Poppycock. His body is adjusting to age just as yours is. Read "His Erection," for some important facts.

If you are a man, you may feel that your partner doesn't love you because she hasn't been having sex with you. This is almost certainly not so, but rather part of the Great Irony of men, women, and sex. In general, men feel loved when their partner has sex with them, and women need to feel loved, safe and cherished to want to have sex.

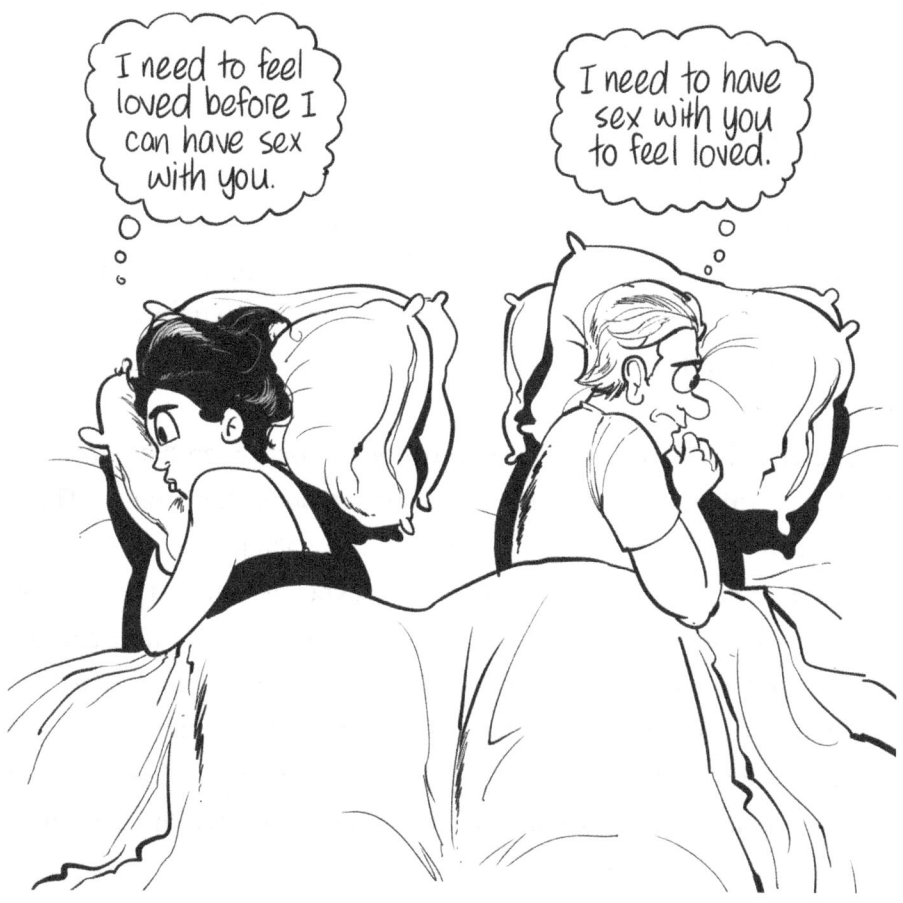

So, if you are a woman and your man isn't paying enough attention to you for you to feel loved, it may be because he's resentful and hurt by what he sees as your lack of love for not having sex with him. It's a vicious cycle. The key is understanding each other. We don't have to be the same, but if we come at it with love and understanding we can find some happy middle ground.

If it has been a very long time, if you feel asexual or "broken," you need to awaken and reconnect with your body. You might start by turning the music up loud when you're alone in the house and dancing, wildly, passionately. As has been proven in dozens of studies, your body tells your mind how to feel. If you make yourself smile, you will feel happier. If you stand more confidently, you will feel more confident. If you dance your own sensual "dance of the seven veils," your body is going to tell you how to feel sensual. Extra points if you do this in the nude.

Exercise is always good, of course. You don't even have to think "exercise," if that word has bad connotations for you. Think "movement." Rock and roll while you are vacuuming. Play some tennis. Really dig into the garden. Maybe even try a little hula hooping—getting those hips swaying in a rhythmic motion might just remind you of some other ways you enjoyed moving that pelvis. Anything to get that body moving and your blood flowing counts. If you lose a few pounds in the effort, so much the better. Exercise will improve your mood, increase your strength and health, and most importantly here, connect you with your body.

Meditation and yoga are other great ways to build a mind-body connection. You don't have to twist yourself up into a pretzel. Just search You Tube for "yoga for seniors" and you will be amazed at the variety of options out there.

Start worshiping your body. Your body is amazing. It truly is a temple. Your body has survived so much, and perhaps even performed the miracle of new life, as well as nourished it. Think about your body and your bits differently, use different words, maybe your own words. See "What Do I Call It?" in the "How to Be Here Now" chapter to learn how important language is to our self-image.

And explore your body. Yes, masturbate. You'll learn plenty about self-love in our chapters on masturbation and sex toys. Lie in a warm, dimly lit or dark room, turn on the music, and touch yourself everywhere. Find out how it feels. Maybe add a few drops of lube to your fingers. Touch your belly, feel your fingers and ears, stroke your breasts and run your hands down your legs. Feel your labia and vagina. Even if you don't climax or even plan on climaxing, touch and learn about yourself. Honor yourself. You are special and beautiful.

If you have trouble getting out of your own head, consider trying a little bit of cannabis. Just a single toke may stop the spinning and self-consciousness and allow you to focus on your own touch and the feelings it awakens.

GETTING IN TOUCH WITH EACH OTHER

When did you stop touching each other? Maybe you didn't want to disturb the kids with overt Public Displays of Affection (PDA). Maybe a distance has grown between you because of hurts and resentments that have built as your sex life faded. Maybe you've just been doing your own things for so long that, now that the kids are gone, you hardly know what to say to one another.

Incendiary sex doesn't happen by itself, but is simply the peak or high point in a deeply sensual and loving relationship. To reach the peak, you need a strong base to build from. For every head-spinning orgasm there needs to be a base of a thousand words and a hundred kisses, hugs and touches. How do you begin to build that base, and get back to the affection you once showed decades ago?

Well, everything starts with Kindness, as you'll hear repeated throughout this book. Read the section on "Kindness." It's hard for anyone, man or woman, to want to be loving and intimate if they feel criticized, disapproved of, disregarded, shamed, or diminished.

Now that you are determined to get in touch with one another again, there are many ways to bring back that daily touch. Here are just a few ideas:

- Do fun things together, dance, walk in the moonlight, find a concert you both want to hear. See an art film or some old black and white classic and talk about it afterwards. Plan a trip together.

- Stop passing each other like ships in the night. Require a kissing toll. Remember, the rugrats aren't watching anymore. There is no one to be embarrassed by how corny this might appear.

- Lay your head in your partner's lap when watching TV. He'll probably naturally stroke your hair.

- Take turns reading this book to one another, and stop and discuss it after each section. Find any book you both enjoy and read to each other.

- Turn that perfunctory good night peck into at least a five-second real kiss.

- Find one fun board game or card game that you can play together.

- Go back to an old make-out spot and reminisce.

- Exercise together, or play physical games—but no heavy competition. This is supposed to be fun!

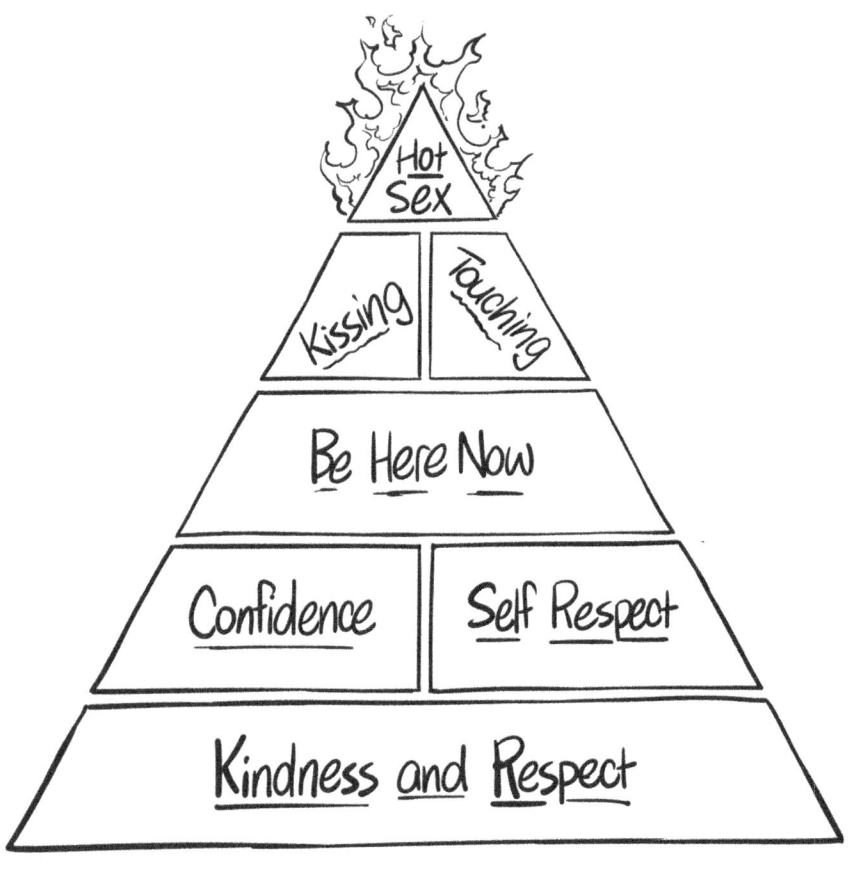

Is talking together going to be awkward after barely communicating all this time? Maybe, but that will fade with time. Great sex doesn't happen in vacuum; it's built on a mountain of kindness and affection.

NAKED TIME — HOW TO GET TO GREAT SEX BY NOT HAVING SEX.

OK, you're talking again and smooching regularly after all these years. You would like to think about sex, but you still have a lot of fears, and you're scared to commit. The answer is: Don't Have Sex.

Decide absolutely, 100 percent, no reservations or slyly winking eyes, that you will not have sex that night. Dim the lights, light the candles, turn on the music and create your total "Be Here Now" space, take your clothes off and snuggle into bed. Maybe have a toke off your favorite vape pen. And then…*do not have sex.*

You can pick the duration. Maybe you'll commit to being naked and focused on each other for an hour together, maybe just half an hour. What are the rules? Just that you focus on each other but won't have sex. However, you get to decide what "Sex" means that night! Maybe any touching of genitals is verboten, but breast, leg, and back massages are in. Perhaps sex only means oral or vaginal sex, and a little mutual masturbation isn't breaking the rules. You decide, but decide *before* you get into bed. The point is to remove the pressure, fears, and expectations, and spend some naked time together touching and kissing.

This way you build up slowly. You learn to be comfortable together again. You can start out with everything involving genitals or ass off limits, and start extending the "in-bounds" areas on successive nights. You may even need to start out wearing clothing if being naked together feels too scary at first. With this slow and measured practice, you can also learn how to create and refine your "Be Here Now" space. Soon, just seeing your ready "Be Here Now" space could start your juices flowing, as could the thought of what you'll do with the new "in-bounds" sexual territory as you progress together.

> ***Sex isn't just intercourse; it's any sexual activity that gives you and your partner pleasure without pain.***

That brings up another issue: redefining what "sex" is (outside of the non-sex sex game we recommended above, where you decide what "sex" is on a given night to protect your boundaries). Bill Clinton thought he could get away with saying "I did not have sexual relations with that woman," because he and Monica Lewinsky only engaged in oral sex and (theoretically at least) never had intercourse. Did anyone buy that? No! Of course oral sex is sex. For that matter, if you give or get a hand job, isn't that sex? What about a totally sensual breast massage?

Senior men will generally take longer to climax than they used to, while post-menopausal women are often more tender and can find prolonged intercourse painful, even though they too need lots of time to build to climax. To keep everyone happy and satisfied, you may need to change it up a bit. Sex isn't just intercourse, it's any sexual activity that gives you and your partner pleasure without pain.

CANNABIS – TAKE AWAY THE TENSION

Do you remember how we started this Chapter of "It's Been a Looong Time"? Let's refresh your memory with some highlights:

- "There is probably no subject more loaded with emotional baggage than sex."
- "It cuts right to the most vulnerable core of us, to our sense of self and our deepest needs and insecurities."
- "Sex is often at the core of the biggest, longest-lasting tensions in a relationship, which can last for decades, sucking life out of an otherwise good relationship."

Heavy, right? How can you even sit together without tension, and without a dozen old arguments playing in your head? Well, if you are lucky enough to be in a state where legal pot is available, there may be a way to break the tension. See all of the sections in "Sex and Cannabis." below. Pot, used judiciously, can not only enhance sex, but it can get couples that normally could barely communicate talking, giggling and making a humongous batch of chocolate chip cookies together.

Give it a try, but read all our sections on Cannabis, as you don't want to have a bad experience. Pot will have different effects on different people, and first-timers may not feel anything at all. But if it works, you may see your mutual tensions just float away like the wispy smoke from your vape pen. And isn't that worth a try?

SEX AND CANNABIS

This is a book on how to connect to your partner and enjoy incendiary sex, regardless of age. Can you have amazing, mind-blowing sex without cannabis? Absolutely. In "How to Be Here Now," we show you many ways that don't involve cannabis to find that special moment when your head stops spinning and your entire world is the taste, touch and scent of your partner.

But cannabis is a useful tool that can help you find that special moment, especially when it's been a long time, or outside stresses make it difficult for you to be in the moment and truly connect with your partner. In this chapter, we will show you the best way of enjoying cannabis with sex in the section "How to Use Cannabis in your Love Life." If this is your first time, or if your last joint was in 1978, you'll want to read "Cannabis, What to Expect the First Time." If you are nervous about trying the "demon weed," read "Cannabis, Good or Bad?" and get the facts. Finally, even if you are familiar with marijuana, if you haven't been to a modern recreational dispensary, you are in for a head-spinning treat. Read "Let's Visit a Dispensary" to help you navigate the dizzying array of new and unfamiliar products and find what will help you the most.

Enjoy the ride.

Without Pot

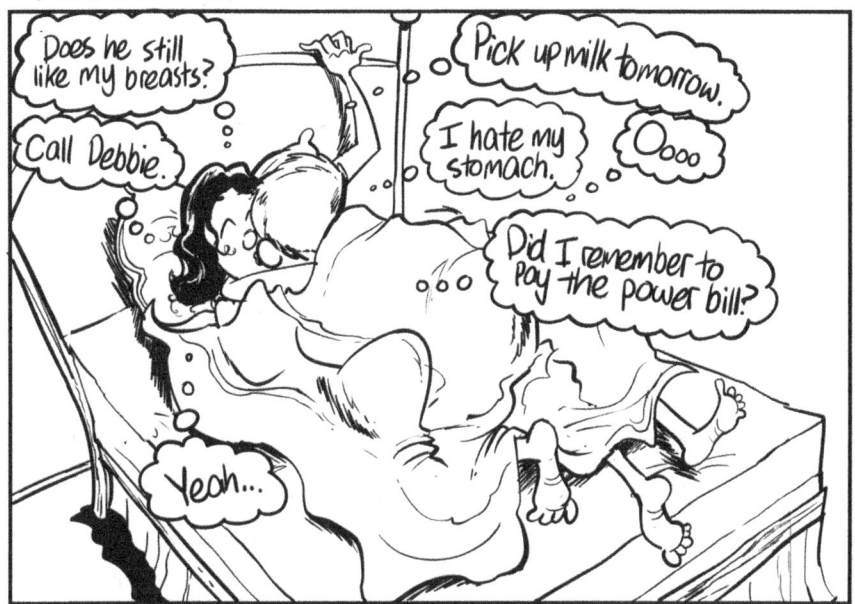

With Pot

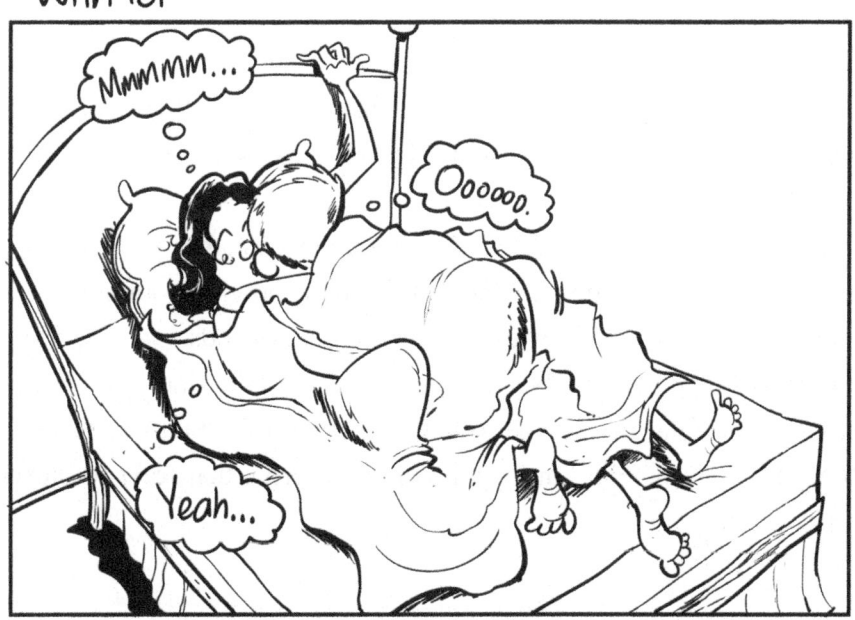

HOW TO USE CANNABIS IN YOUR LOVE LIFE

Is there anything loaded with more baggage than sex? It cuts to the most vulnerable core of us. As you begin to take off your clothes, anxieties over your body, your performance, and what's in your partner's mind vie in your head with the normal swirl of concerns over money, children, and household repairs. Is it any wonder that it's hard to let go of everything except the enjoyment of the moment and to "Be Here Now"?

This is where cannabis can help. Used right, cannabis can help stop the swirl in your head, and at the same time increase your awareness of the sensations of taste and touch and help you and your partner connect with kindness and empathy. Used wrong, it can lead to anxiety and the stoned inability to follow complex sentences. Let us help you use it correctly.

First, some basic terminology. Back in the day, there was pretty much one form of pot which was referred to as "bud," "weed," "Mary Jane," "Scooby Doo," or a plethora of other names, but it was all the same thing. This is the dried flower of the cannabis plant that you crushed up and rolled into a joint or stuck in the bowl of your bong. (For those of you who somehow missed this boat in the 60s and 70s, a bong is a form of pipe that involves using water to cool the smoke as it passes through, allowing the smoke to get deeper into the lungs.) That was then, this is now. Here are some common terms that refer to current forms of pot:

- **Flower:** This is the modern term for the old-school bud. This is the dried plant that you would smoke the old-fashioned way. This is probably the most economical way to get your pot, but smoking a joint or using a pipe or bong does tend to burn the throat, especially for the neophyte pot-smoker.

- **Vaporizers or Vape Pens:** With these, you are getting a concentrated oil from the cannabis plant and then inhaling it through the use of a vaporizing device that instantly heats the oil and turns it into a sort of mist that you suck in through one end of the device. This is a virtually odorless version of smoking, which makes it ideal for using indoors (i.e., right in bed). It is significantly less harsh on the throat, and there are no ashes of any kind to deal with. The effects can be felt almost immediately, and typically last an hour to a few hours.

These devices are sometimes called vape pens because they look sort of like small pens. These come in several varieties, but in general there are two categories: reusable and disposable. The reusable ones have two parts: the battery and heating device, and cartridges with the pot oil that you attach to the device, replacing as needed. The disposable vape pens are the full package: they have both the concentrated oil and the heating device all in one and are meant to be used until the oil is gone and then thrown away.

Complete detailed instructions on use of the XS-2000B Disposable Vape Pen...

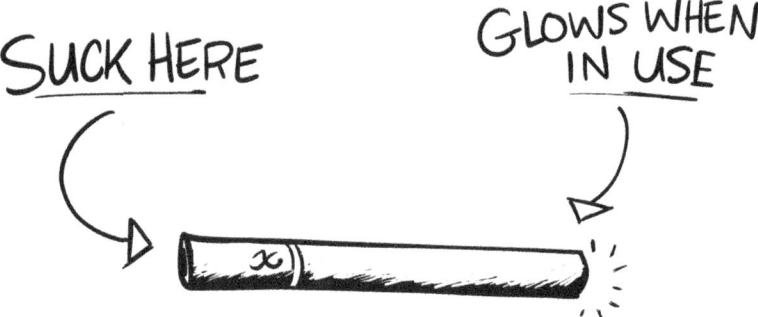

- **Edibles:** This is the modern-day version of the classic pot brownie. Only now it is more likely to look like a designer chocolate truffle or a package of gummy bears. Although the term "edibles" implies this is pot mixed into something you eat, this also covers liquid forms such as pot-laced root beer or lemonade. When you smoke pot, it enters your system very quickly through your lungs and into the blood stream. When you eat the pot, it has to first get processed through your digestive system before anything really gets into your blood stream. As we will discuss in greater length below, these yummy looking treats can be very tempting, but it is extremely hard to properly dose yourself because there is such a long delay between ingestion and the effects of the ingestion—sometimes several hours. And while the effects from smoking or vaping pot usually last an hour or two, the effects from edibles can last significantly longer.

- **THC:** This stands for tetrahydrocannabinol, which is the compound found in pot that makes you experience a "high."

- **Indica, Sativa and Hybrid:** These terms refer to the strain of cannabis plant where the flower or oil came from. Indica tends to produce feelings of mental and physical relaxation and can provide pain relief. This strain is usually intended for evening use. Sativa can be used to address feelings of depression and anxiety, to treat chronic pain and increase focus and creativity. It is more stimulating than Indica so it is generally recommended that it be used during the day. A hybrid of the two can theoretically give you the best of both worlds.

- **Terpenes:** These are aromatic organic hydrocarbons found in cannabis that are responsible for a given strain's taste and smell, and can modify the effects of THC.

OK, back to the discussion about incorporating pot into your sex life. When do you use it during sex? Make it part of foreplay, or even make it a little ceremony as part of the start of an evening (or afternoon, or morning) adventure. You might each have a single toke to unwind. Especially if it's a vape or flower with a high percentage of THC, a single toke—or even a half toke—may be all you need to stop the swirl in your head. Snuggle together for five minutes or so. If the swirl in your head hasn't stopped swirling, you could try another toke, but be careful, the quickest way to have a bad experience is to take too much.

As you'll read in "What to Expect the First Time," if you've never used cannabis, it's very common not to feel the effects the first time. So, perhaps the first time or two if you don't feel any effects, just let it go and make the best of your time with your lover. Don't keep taking hits assuming you just haven't had enough.

It's best if both partners try a little together, or at least that the partner who isn't partaking is fully on board with the experiment. It goes without saying that you never, never, try to get someone high without their knowledge and consent. That's probably illegal, and if it isn't, it should be.

It also goes without saying that when under the influence you should never drive, operate machinery, or be in any environment that would not be totally safe for a hyperactive toddler. Be sure you are where you plan to be for the rest of the day or night. You may not know how long the high feeling will last, especially those first several times you try it. Reserve this experiment for when you are home and expect to stay home for at least the next eight hours.

What form of cannabis should you use? We recommend that you start with either a disposable vape or flower in either Indica or hybrid. Avoid edibles until you really understand the issues with edibles. Read "Let's Visit a Dispensary" for all the details.

How much should you take? Very, very, little. Start with one toke (one hit), and only consider another toke if after 5 minutes the swirl in your head hasn't started to subside. While you may have fantastic sex on a lot of pot, too much can also lead to bad experiences. The amount that it takes to help you "Be Here Now" is often much less than someone would use to just "get high." Also, if you have great sex, you want to remember it, right? At our age "getting lucky" can mean walking into a room and remembering why you came in there. So, add that to being stoned on pot along with the standard PCBs (Post-Coital Brainlessness), and you may find that you lose all memories of the greatest sex of your life—and possibly your ability to understand the English language.

We've found there is a very fine line between the right amount to make us feel present and ready for some great sex and the amount that makes us feel stoned and shut off from our bodies to the point where we have no interest in having sex. This is the "bi-modal effect" paradox. The effects of a smaller dose can be diametrically opposite to the effects of a larger dose.

What will it feel like? Even if it's not your first time using cannabis, read "What to Expect the First Time," to remind yourself of how variable the experience can be and what you might expect. In fact, read it even if you've been a casual user over the years, because very few of us ever read a "How To" guide on using cannabis, and you might learn a few things! At its best, by adding cannabis to your lovemaking you can enter an ethereal and joyous world where time slows, sensations heighten, and the cares and thoughts of the world have evaporated as you ascend to new heights.

However, here is a final warning. While pot is not physically addictive like many prescription drugs, alcohol or nicotine are, that doesn't mean that it can't harm you if you have a tendency for addiction. After all, there is nothing physically addictive about food or gambling, but that hasn't stopped many people from abusing them and hurting themselves and their loved ones in the process. What we are advocating here is the very judicious use of a small amount of pot every now and then. If you know you are someone prone to over-do when it comes to substance use, you may need to sit this one out.

WHAT TO EXPECT THE FIRST TIME

We'll go out on a limb and suggest that this is perhaps the first time you've read a manual on how to use pot, right? Probably the most education any of us received in the past was a reminder to put our finger over the airhole when sucking on a bong, or perhaps to keep Visine handy so Mom wouldn't see our red eyes.

You can have wonderful experiences with cannabis, and also not-so-wonderful experiences. Below you will find advice and tips to help make sure your experience is the former, not the latter.

- You need to inhale. Bill Clinton was doing it wrong! It may seem obvious, but some people will pull the vapor or smoke into their mouths and not their lungs, and wonder why nothing happens. Suck in the smoke or vapor and hold it. Try to keep it in for about five seconds or so and then exhale. If you are taking tiny hits to avoid coughing or just because that's all you want, continue to breath air in fully after the tiny hit, to make sure the smoke or vapor goes into the lungs and bloodstream, rather than staying in your throat.

- Coughing. When you breath in the smoke or vapor, it may feel like it expands in your lungs and can cause a coughing jag, which is not fun at all. Until you are used to it, take in only very tiny amounts at a time. It's good to have a glass of water handy to cool the throat. Several small hits will have the same effect as one larger one so there is no reason to push things.

- Be prepared to not get high. A survey found that 41 percent of first time users did not feel the effects, and another 13 percent were not sure. Your brain may not have enough receptors for the cannabinoids, but it will make more by the time you try it again. Many people don't have a great experience the first time. Dust yourself off and try again another day.

- Have plenty of water and snacks at hand. (While there is a common stereotype that pot gives you "the munchies," this is not actually very likely to happen in the small quantities we are recommending here.)

- Make sure there is nothing you "have" to do. Make sure you won't be interrupted. Consider turning off your phone.

- Do not watch a scary movie while high. You have more empathy for the characters, and you feel more a part of the action. Take our advice here.

- What if I'm too high? First, remember this will only typically last a few hours. Turn on the tube and connect with the couch. Also, many people find drinking a cup of coffee or biting on peppercorns will "kill" the high.

- How long does it last? If you are using modest amounts of a vape pen or flower, the effect usually lasts about 1 to 3 hours, but that can vary, and some people (such as Julia) can find that it may last longer on certain nights. Edibles are another story, and the high can last 12 hours or more. (See "Let's Visit a Dispensary" for the full story.)

If you get high—in a good way—you might experience any or all of the following effects:

- You may feel euphoric, uplifted.
- Everything becomes funny, and you may not be able to stop laughing.
- Your senses may become heightened. You may experience touch, taste and color more strongly. You may find your partner's touch like you've never felt it and find your entire skin is now an erogenous zone.
- You may get "The Munchies." Have plenty of food and drink easily at hand. You can't drive to the store for ice cream, so think ahead. (But see our note above about small amounts of pot not being likely to cause this side-effect.)
- You feel physically at ease. If you were nauseous, that feeling will generally go away, which is why people undergoing cancer treatments find pot so helpful.
- Time gets funny. Time may seem to stretch out, with 20 minutes feeling like an hour's experience.
- You open up and become more empathetic. You could find yourself getting into deep, intimate discussions and bonding with your partner.
- You become profound (or at least you may think you are). You may see the deep connections and meaning between all objects in the universe. Some of this is real. Artists of all kinds have used cannabis to think creatively and see things in

new ways. But don't be surprised if you write down your world-changing thoughts, and on reading them the next day go "Huh?"

- You may feel horny. The loss of self-consciousness, feelings of empathy and connection, and increased sensations of touch and taste may kick up your sex drive.

If you get high—in a bad way—usually by taking too much or being in a bad environment, you might experience any or all of the following. Remember, the effect will go away in a few hours. Turn on a comedy.

- Anxiety and paranoia. You can get frightened of your surroundings, or fearful of interacting with anyone.
- Sadness.
- Physical discomfort.
- Confusion.
- Reduced sex drive. Ironic isn't it? A little can make you horny, but too much can kill your sex drive, even if you were ready for play.
- Inability to follow even simple conversations.

If you do not have a good experience, try to understand why. Was it the environment? Did you take too much? Was it the wrong variety? A strong Sativa can be wonderful, but can also bring on anxiety and paranoia in some people. If you didn't feel anything, just try again another day. If, in the end, Cannabis isn't for you, don't worry. This is just one tool that helps some people "Be Here Now." You can have mind-blowing, incendiary sex perfectly well without it. Read "Being Here Now" and "Mating Rituals," and find what works for you.

CANNABIS: GOOD OR BAD?

While we're sure we can all agree sex is good for you, what about cannabis? With the millions of pages that have been written about the "demon weed," it is understandable that you may have concerns about ingesting something that for most of our lives has been illegal and often demonized. What is the truth? Here we try to synopsize the health and legal issues around pot.

OK, first the bad. Even though at the time of this writing 30 states have legalized marijuana for medical use, and 9 states and Canada have legalized it for recreational use, marijuana is still listed federally as a Schedule I controlled substance. This means that it would be very unwise to take your recreational dispensary purchases across state lines. Additionally, because of its status as a controlled substance, it has been difficult to do medical studies on cannabis, and its effects are less studied than those of alcohol and tobacco.

Smoking in any context, whether cannabis, tobacco, or sitting around a campfire is not ideal for your lungs. Using a vape, as we recommend, instead of directly smoking will reduce but not eliminate any respiratory risks associated with cannabis. Some studies suggest that heavy adolescent use of cannabis can affect their growing brains, and even reduce their I.Q. by the time they are adults.

> *"The Nixon campaign in 1968, and the Nixon White House after that, had two enemies: the antiwar left and black people. You understand what I'm saying? We knew we*

couldn't make it illegal to be either against the war or black, but by getting the public to associate the hippies with marijuana and blacks with heroin, and then criminalizing both heavily, we could disrupt those communities. We could arrest their leaders, raid their homes, break up their meetings, and vilify them night after night on the evening news. Did we know we were lying about the drugs? Of course we did." John Erlichman – Counselor to President Richard Nixon, 1994 interview

Now for the better news. On the legal front, the tide is turning. Legislators on both sides of the aisle are pushing for removing pot from the Schedule I list, and decriminalizing or legalizing it's use. Public opinion has shifted dramatically and a strong majority of both Democrats and Republicans now support legalization. John Boehner, a conservative republican and former Speaker of the House who was "unalterably opposed" to marijuana legalization is now on the board of a cannabis growing company, and touts its ability to reduce chronic pain and to help reverse the opioid epidemic.

Cannabis was not always demonized, as it has been for most of our lives. In fact, taking a toke puts you in some pretty fine company!

George Washington. Yes, the father of our country was likely the first presidential toker. He advocated the growing of hemp for industrial use, and many believe that he used the female flower of his hemp plants to relieve his toothaches. We're not casting aspersions on such an icon. A total of 11 presidents, including John Adams, Thomas Jefferson,

James Madison, James Monroe, Andrew Jackson, Zachary Taylor, Franklin Pierce, John F. Kennedy, Bill Clinton, George W. Bush and Barack Obama, are believed to have lit up from time to time.

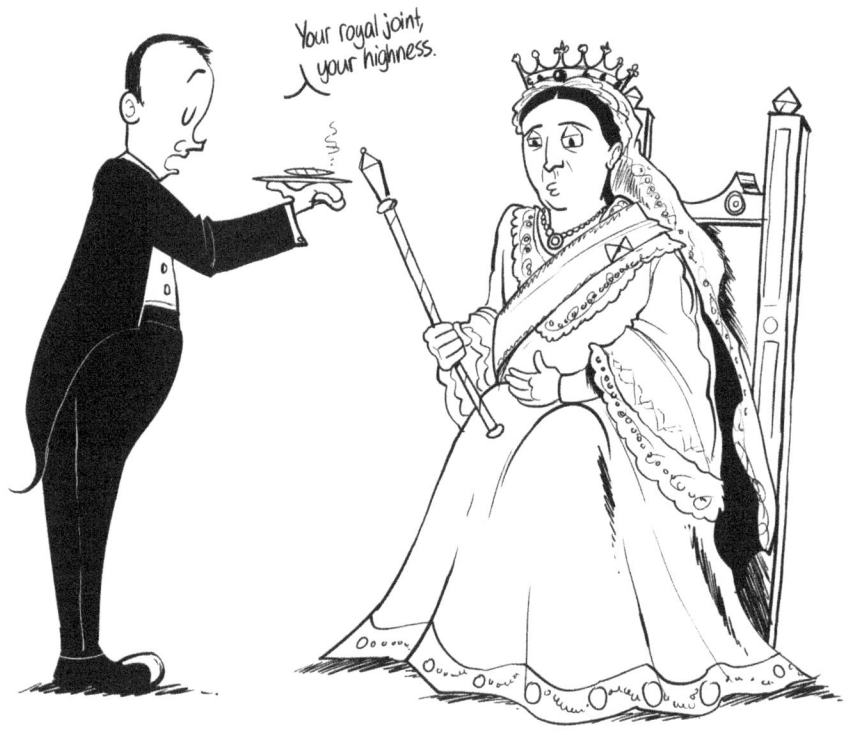

Queen Victoria. Yes, she who ruled Britain from 1837 until 1901, back when the "Sun Never Sets on the British Empire," used marijuana to reduce the pain of menstrual cramps. Her personal physician Sir J.

Russell Reynolds wrote in 1890 that "When pure and administered carefully, [cannabis] is one of the most valuable medicines we possess."

Louisa May Alcott. The author of "Little Women" wrote many short pieces on pot, including the "Perilous Play," where two lovers get high, get lost in a boat, and then get engaged in the last act. One of her stories ends with the line "Heaven Bless Hashish."

William Shakespeare. OK, we don't know for sure, but historians found clay pipes in Shakespeare's house with traces of marijuana in them that date from his residence. Why else would he pen a sonnet about the "noted weed"?

Carl Sagan and Francis Crick. Does marijuana harm the intellect? Well, the celebrated Mr. "Billions and Billions of years ago," and the Nobel prize winning co-discoverer of DNA didn't seem to think so. In the height of the marijuana prohibition in 1971 Carl Sagan wrote an article under the pseudonym "Mr. X," talking about the positive influence of pot to his personal and professional life.

Margaret Mead, Maya Angelou and Isak Dinensen (a.k.a. Karen Blixen). Margaret Mead, the famous anthropologist, got into serious hot water in 1969 for advocating the legalization of pot to the US Senate.

[Michael] *So, given the notable Presidents, authors and scientists who have enjoyed cannabis, it's hard to argue that taking a toke is going to make you a bad person. I like to imagine a scene where all these people are sitting around a campfire, passing around a joint and getting high. Put me right down between Carl Sagan and Francis Crick please.*

Can you imagine the spacey and mind-blowing conversation that would ensue?

On the health side, cannabis has been shown in studies to reduce chronic pain, including arthritis pain, reduce the potential for seizures, increase appetite, reduce anxiety (in low doses), and reduce muscle spasms. Some studies even suggest it can slow the progress of Alzheimer's disease and cancer. Like all studies, you should take these with a grain of salt, but it seems clear that there are some benefits and relatively little harm in light cannabis use. In fact, a 2015 report published in the respected journal "Nature" comparing the risks of cannabis to tobacco, alcohol and several other drugs found that cannabis represented the lowest risk of all by large margins.[9]

Finally, we have found that when combining cannabis and sex, the best effects occur with very low doses and infrequent use. "Everything in moderation" is a good guide to go by.

> **When combining cannabis and sex, the best effects occur with very low doses and infrequent use.**

[Julia] *Like a lot of people, my early experiences with pot dated back to high school and college. I had never purchased any, but I did smoke every now and then if a friend offered. I could probably count on two hands the number of times this happened. It basically made me hungry*

---

[9] https://www.nature.com/articles/srep08126

and tired, two things that I wasn't super anxious to feel as I got older. The thought of buying something illegal from some sketchy kid on a street corner and coming home with a baggy that could contain literally anything felt creepy and even dangerous. Not to mention the smell, the red eyes, and the cotton mouth. None of this made me want to turn into a regular pot head.

After Michael and I got together he told me that he still liked to smoke pot from time to time. I had no interest in joining him, and quite honestly felt it was a little childish of him to still imbibe. It seemed to me he should have grown out of that phase by now. Although I felt that using marijuana seemed like a somewhat juvenile way to "chill out," I had no similar value judgments about someone who liked to have a glass of wine in the evenings to relax and come down after a long day.

After Colorado passed the first recreational pot law in 2012 (which went into effect in January of 2014), I realized there was no logical reason to think about pot as something all that different from the way I view alcohol. They are both legal substances that can be enjoyed by consenting adults. And in moderation, both can help you relax and be a little more social. I also realized that alcohol has a much greater propensity for harm than marijuana does. People are more likely to have an addiction problem with alcohol than with pot, and when someone is drunk, they can become abusive and seriously dangerous.

"Alcohol, more than any illegal drug, was found to be closely associated with violent crimes, including murder, rape, assault, child and spousal abuse. About 3 million violent crimes occur each year in which victims perceive the offender to have been drinking and statistics

related to alcohol use by violent offenders generally show that about half of all homicides and assaults are committed when the offender, victim, or both have been drinking. Among violent crimes, with the exception of robberies, the offender is far more likely to have been drinking than under the influence of other drugs." The National Council on Alcoholism and Drug Dependence, Inc.[10]

I realized my value judgment about pot really made no sense from a logical perspective. Add to that the fact that new technologies have made the most negative aspects of using pot a thing of the past. With the new vape pens, you can now get the benefits of the high without stinking up your clothes, your hair and your house, and without the other negative side effects such as red eyes and dry mouth. I opened up to the possibility that maybe there was something positive I could get from trying pot once again.

It took some trial and error, but I now know that my preferred method of imbibing is to use a disposable vape pen, and that I can take just a hit or two and I will almost instantly feel relaxed and calm and present. With such a low dosage, I don't feel tired and it does not give me the "munchies" either.

Opening myself to marijuana has been a huge boost to our sex life because on those days where we want some romance but can't seem to shut off the mental chatter, we share a hit or two of our favorite vape pen and the noise of the day just melts away. We can connect and be

---

[10] *www.ncadd.org/about-addition/alcohol-drugs-and-crime*

present. It is hot, sexy and amazing when the mental tapes stop playing and you can just "Be Here Now" with your lover.

The key, we've found, is both finding the right strain of pot and using the right amount. Too much will make you feel spacy and sort of shutdown. They call this the bi-modal effect. One dose can make you feel energized and alive, and another can have the exact opposite effect. So toss your old value judgments aside, start very slowly, and see if you can't find just the right dose to kick your sex-life up a notch!

LET'S VISIT A DISPENSARY

So, pot is legal in your state, or maybe you've taken a road trip out to the West Coast and stared amazed as you drive by billboards advertising weed and pass shops with green crosses and names like "StarBuds." Perhaps you remember buying weed, nervously passed in a baggie in the back seat of a Chevy, or listening to Cheech and Chong, and remembering that time your friend made a pipe out of a potato and aluminum foil. Maybe you've never toked in your life, or had that one hit on a joint at a party in 1976.

Well, things have changed, and for the better. Here we are going to give you the 50+ Seniors' Introduction to Legal Pot Products and Dispensaries. If you are fairly new to dispensaries and are considering using it as we describe in this book—infrequently in small doses to enhance your lovemaking—then you will want to read this, as the advice you may get at the dispensary itself isn't really designed for you. On the other hand, if you're a regular cannabis consumer who buys in ounces and knows what "dabbing" is, then perhaps you can move on, and please don't write us long letters on the essential flavor and effect differences of the terpenes found in "Sour Diesel" versus "Golden Goat."

Prepare to be amazed. Pot is now an Industry with a capital "I." According to a Forbes Magazine article published in March 2018, spending on legal cannabis worldwide is expected to hit $57 billion by 2027. The array of products available today bears as much resemblance to that little baggie of weed as your iPhone does to the old dial telephone that was tethered to the wall in your parent's kitchen. OK, let's assume that you've read the "Sex and Cannabis" chapter, and you're considering entering this new weird world. Here we go.

Pot shops or legal marijuana dispensaries vary widely. About the only common thing is that you will show your driver's license when you enter, regardless of how old you look, and probably again when you buy something, even if it's the same guy who just saw your license two minutes ago. Also, don't forget to bring cash. Until Federal laws catch up, all dispensaries are cash-only businesses. (Many even have ATM machines right inside for this reason.)

You may find that some dispensaries are pungent places with heavily tattooed twenty-somethings presiding over bell jars of green buds and a line of glass bongs on the back wall. On the other hand, upon entering other dispensaries you may feel that you've stumbled into an Apple store by accident, gleaming white and chrome with colorful display cases and free espresso while you wait to be served. They have frequent buyer programs and daily specials. The "Budmeister" or "Budtender" that serves you might be a young woman with tattoos, orange hair and a collection of piercings, or a grandma in a sweater she knitted herself. Almost everyone is happy, relaxed and helpful, and the people working the counter are usually cannabis enthusiasts who are most used to serving medical marijuana users and other cannabis enthusiasts. Which is why, if you are the intended audience for this section they could—with the best of intentions—steer you wrong.

Below are a few of our opinions, and opinions vary widely. As well, effects vary from person to person, so what works for you may not work for your partner. Also, used as we suggest, this is really inexpensive. A disposable vape pen may cost $35, but could last you and your partner through five and maybe even ten or more sex sessions, making it less expensive per session than a single glass of wine, split between the two of you. So while it may be economical to buy in bulk, we recommend you buy single use disposable vape pens or single grams of flower and experiment, as there is no reason to worry about economy until you find what works for the two of you.

Sativa, Indica or Hybrid? Cannabis Sativa and Cannibis Indica are the two species of Cannabis used in recreational marijuana. Hybrid is, as previously noted, a hybrid between the two. These are the three primary classes you will often find in a dispensary, and one of the first questions a Budmeister might ask you is your preference between them. Generally, Sativa strains are considered to provide a "head" or "cerebral" high, energizing and uplifting. Indica strains are believed to be more of a "body" high, relaxing, calming, even sedating. Hybrid strains are somewhere in between.

However, these are just generalities. There are over 100 different compounds and terpenes within cannabis that can alter the effect, so not every Indica is relaxing, and not every Sativa is energizing. And for the cognoscenti, the three categories are not nearly discriminating enough. Marijuana enthusiasts may describe their favorite flower with as complex a set of adjectives as a wine steward.

However, to start out we recommend either an Indica or hybrid. Sativa can be very enjoyable, but the energizing effect can turn to anxiousness and even paranoia in some people—definitely not what you are trying for in a lovemaking enhancer. On the other hand, some people will be so relaxed on Indica that they fall asleep.

The other primary choice is the ratio of THC to CBD in the product you buy. THC and CBD are just two of the roughly 100 compounds in pot, but are the two primary ones you might discuss at a dispensary. THC is the primary psychoactive compound in marijuana. It's what makes you hungry and high, may increase sensations and taste, and can relieve pain and nausea. CBD is a non-intoxicating compound that can help with anxiety, pain and inflammation. THC or CBD will be described as a concentration in the cannabis product, or as a ratio between them, as in 2:1 THC to CBD.

For lovemaking, we find the most beneficial effect of cannabis is relaxing you and stopping the spinning in your head, the thousand thoughts that keep you from Being Here Now. Strains that are 100 percent CBD have many important medical qualities, but these have not been effective, at least for us, for lovemaking purposes. A CBD-dominant mixture of CBD and THC can be very good, but would not be a good one to use if you are already tired, as you may drift off before the night gets going. In general, we'd recommend either pure THC or THC to CBD ratios of no more than 1:1. Again, your experience may vary.

You may also hear about terpenes from your Budmeister. Terpenes are aromatic compounds produced by many fruits and flowers. In cannabis, terpenes are flavor compounds that may also alter the intoxicating effect in different ways. Think "aromatherapy" here. In aromatherapy, certain aromas will energize or relax you, and different terpenes in cannabis will do the same. However, the "aroma" is the widely varying scent of pot, which some may enjoy, and others not. So, when your Budmiester recommends a vape pen because it has interesting terpenes, remember he is talking about different pot flavors, and the modifying effects of the terpenes on the experience. If you want it to smell lightly of cherries or pumpkin spice, then buy that. If you want your vape exhalation to smell more like pot (but also perhaps have slightly different effects from pure THC), then get the ones with terpenes. Within the classes of Indica, Sativa and hybrid, growers have created a huge suite of different varieties with inventive names, all with different combinations of terpenes.

Now to delivery systems—how you get the THC and/or CBD into your system, ranked in rough order of recommendation.

Our #1 recommendation: Disposable vape pens. This is by far the easiest, least complicated and least smelly way to use cannabis for lovemaking, and also the easiest to hide from the kids (or aging parents you may be caring for). A disposable vape pen is a cigarette-sized tube that contains concentrated cannabis oil and an internal battery system. The battery instantly heats the oil and produces a vapor when you suck on one end. It's really that simple. You don't need to assemble anything or charge anything or even push any buttons. You simply suck in on one end.

Most of the models we have tried are almost little works of art, with cool logos and a colored light at the non-inhalation end of the pen. The light is illuminated when you suck in, showing you the pen is working. Vaping also has the advantage of being very quick. You will usually feel the effect in seconds to a few minutes. That way you can control how much you take very easily. They are discreet, they do not create any ash or smoke, and are virtually odorless, which means you can use them indoors without any worries.

Now, aside from disposable vape pens, there are all kinds of reusable vape systems that allow you to load cartridges of your favorite concentrate onto the battery system. Some of these need to be assembled, and some have complicated light patterns to help you select levels of heating or identify how much battery life you have remaining. (Try remembering how that works when you are stoned…) Some even have accompanying iPhone apps to control them. Your Budmeister may point out—truthfully—that the vape systems and cartridges are more cost-effective than the disposable vape pens in the long run, but unless you are a true enthusiast, the cost difference will be minor and in general doesn't beat the convenience of disposal vapes. Remember, your goal here is not to get stoned. A little goes a long way. You are just looking to take the edge off, so arguments about economies of scale don't really make much sense.

As we have said many times, the effect can vary from time to time, even with the same device. We have found that with disposable vapes, the first few hits are often stronger than after we've had a dozen hits on the same pen. Just wait a few minutes between hits, and gauge your level of relaxation before you consider the next one.

Our #2 recommendation: Flower, or what we used to just call pot. There is a rebranding of the actual marijuana bud that we used to call "pot" or "weed" or "Mary Jane" into "flower." It's a nice name and accurate, as this is actually the flower of the marijuana plant. Here's the downside, you have to smoke it, and if you are not used to smoking doing so can be harsh on your throat and may even start a coughing jag (take very little tokes). Also, it smells like, well, pot. You probably won't want to do this inside your house so you have to plan the pot portion of your evening for before you are in your bedroom and undressed.

The upside is that there are many more varieties of flower, so you can customize your experience more precisely based on the specific strain and the combination of terpenes it has. There are even articles on the specific strains of pot that are best for sex, matching different kinds of sex to different strains. By contrast, the purified resins in vape pens have very few terpenes, and are usually just sold as one of three varieties: Indica, Sativa or a hybrid of the two. Like vaping, the effect of smoking flower is quick to come on and will generally only last a few hours. While different strains reviewed for sex effects sounds great, there is no assurance that the "Purple Princess" strain that you read about is actually the same "Purple Princess" strain you have at your local dispensary. With that caveat in mind, here is a list of strains that others have found particularly enhancing for sex:

- Asian fantasy
- Atomic Northern Lights
- Chocolate Chunk
- Danky Doodle
- Flo
- Granddaddy Purple
- Green Crack

- Hindu Skunk
- Purple Princess
- Sour Dream
- Super Sour Diesel
- Ultimate Trainwreck
- Yumbolt
- Lavender Trainwreck
- Cinderella
- Super Lemon Haze

Our #3 recommendation: Vaginal weed lubes. Actually, we haven't been able to make these work for us well, but apparently for many women the effect is glorious. Foria (www.foira.com) is leading the way by providing a coconut-based cannabis spray that is applied directly to the vagina, clitoris and labia. This is then absorbed by your body, and when applied 15 minutes to an hour before playtime can lead to easier or extra-powerful orgasms. Our hesitation is the same as for the edibles we describe below: that an older woman's body has a lower metabolism than a younger woman's, and the absorption and effect may take much longer than the 15 minutes to an hour they recommend. We don't know if it will work for you, but we at least like the idea of a cannabis product specifically made to enhance sex.

Our #4 recommendation: Edibles. You will be very tempted. A good dispensary may have an enormous variety of edibles. The old standard pot brownie has given way to luscious chocolates of all kinds in gorgeous wrappings, lemon drops and mints, baked goods, tasty drinks, teas and much more. Also in this class are sub-lingual drops and tinctures that are meant to be dripped under the tongue.

Generally, most people feel there is often a big difference between the effect you feel on vape or flower versus an edible, but that doesn't necessarily mean the edible experience is not enjoyable, or that it's not good for lovemaking. Our warning is this: your Budmeister may say that you will feel the effects in "30 minutes to an hour" or maybe "one to two hours." He or she may tout sublingual drops which act within "10 to 30 minutes," much quicker than other edibles. Don't believe them.

While what the Budmeister says may be true for a 22-year-old girl with a high metabolism, it will not work the same way for a 66-year-old woman. The time it may take you to feel the effects could be several hours, especially if taken with or after other food. You could take it at 8 p.m., for example, and feel nothing all evening, and later wake up in the middle of the night high. It is difficult to dose, because you won't know the effect *for hours*, and so it's easy to get too high by eating just one more piece of that tasty chocolate edible. Also, **the effect can last 12 hours or more**, and you could easily wake up still stoned. Edibles can be fun and the array of products is astounding, but take care, especially if you have not had much experience with cannabis.

Last and probably least: everything else. So, the list doesn't end there. There are a wide variety of various forms of concentrates, hash oil, "shatter," ICE, BHO, and waxes. There are also topical oils for rubbing on your skin, and pre-made joints, either "pre-rolls" or "blunts." In our minds these are more for enthusiasts. As you read in "Cannabis and Sex," the point for us is not getting stoned, but getting sensual and falling into that timeless moment where the world recedes, and we are the only two people in the world, riding toward heaven. Getting there generally only takes a smidgen of cannabis, and this is one of those cases where more is definitely not better.

HOW TO BE HERE NOW

Today is the age of multitasking. Thousands of things compete for our attention every day. Most jobs today are a welter of small details which we are expected to skillfully juggle, while at the same time being interrupted with a constant stream of incoming emails and texts. Every Web page we visit has ads and article titles screaming, "Click me! Click me!"

This aspect of modern life is rewiring our brains and making it harder and harder to concentrate and focus on any one thing. Remember when they used to say that you needed to "stop and smell the roses"? That sounds so anachronistic in today's frantic environment, but it's never been more apropos.

What were the best moments in your life? What were your happiest times? Think back. Were they moments when your mind was cluttered with an ever-changing To Do list, or were you living the moment, savoring the sensations, simply Being There?

We bet that it was the latter. Here is a key to a happier life: you don't have to wait for those wonderful moments to appear. You can create them. The key to incendiary, mind-blowing sex, or for that matter for the best moments of life in general, is to Be Here Now.

Our daily lives today are broken into thousands of little bite-sized Tweets, our smart phones on our hip, our heightened senses tensed for the next "ding" of an incoming text or Facebook alert. It is any wonder that it's harder today than ever before to just Be Here Now?

But you can. You can create more of those best moments in life, and we want to help you do that. Read on. Try our tips and strategies, explore a few "Mating Rituals," take what we can teach you and add your own flavors and ideas. Be happier. Be Here Now.

TURN ON THE ONS, TURN OFF THE OFFS

When you think back on some of your best sexual times, what one thing do they all have in common? We are guessing that regardless of where you were or who you were with, the common denominator for all these intensely blissful times was that you were completely present with your experience. When sex is really good, everything else seems to disappear. This is what we mean when we say Be Here Now.

In her ground-breaking book, "Come as You Are, The Surprising New Science That Will Transform Your Sex Life," Dr. Emily Nagoski discusses the "dual control model of sexual response." These are the accelerators and the brakes affecting our sex drive—the things that help turn us on and the things that end up turning us off. If you can take the time to identify what some of these things are for you, you will be well on your way to romantic bliss. The key is to "turn on the ons and turn off the offs."

If your mind is cluttered with your To Do list, or you are worried that your underarms smell, or you can't stop thinking about that project you need to complete for work, it will be very challenging for you to get sexually turned on because your brakes are working harder than your accelerator possibly can. Likewise, if it has been a long time since you and your partner had sex, or you are feeling insecure about how your body looks to your lover, it will be very difficult to get out of your head and into the moment.

Instead of getting lost in the sensations, you will find your mind mentally narrating your experience to you. "Now he is kissing my breasts and making his way down my body. Oh God, my belly is so flabby I hope it doesn't disgust him! He is going to go down on me, isn't he? I wish I had showered before going to bed tonight." You get the idea. Can you think of anything less conducive to pure sexual desire?

We have been on a bit of a journey to try to discover the best solutions for turning on the ons and turning off the offs. And we are happy to share these discoveries with you in the sections that follow. What worked for us may or may not work for you, but hopefully these ideas will inspire you to come up with your own custom set of rituals.

SETTING THE STAGE

When we were younger, it didn't take much to set the stage for sex. Heck, the back seat of a car could do the trick. An hour break between classes? Perfect! Basically, if we were both in bed (or the back of a van, or behind a bush in the backyard, or in the office when everyone had already left) at the same time and some part of our bodies happened to touch, one thing would inevitably lead to another.

Between decreased hormones and energy levels, and potentially *decades* with the same sexual partner, those magical spontaneous moments are a thing of the past. If we want to reignite the sexual fire, we need to put a little more effort into the mix at this stage of our lives. But when we say effort, we don't want you to think of this as another chore on your To Do list. Instead, think in terms of setting an *intention,* an *expectation.* The time you take to transform your space, cleanse your body and physically and emotionally shut the rest of the world out are not just preludes to romance but very critical forms of foreplay.

In fact, if you get into a "romance ritual" along the lines of what we suggest below, you might discover that simply turning on the special sex music or lighting the candles will start to trigger your body's arousal response. Remember Pavlov from your Psych 101 class? He's the guy who rang a bell immediately before feeding his dogs each day. After a while, the mere sound of the bell got the dogs salivating. That anticipation of good things to come is what we are talking about here.

Expectation and anticipation. Places and events create emotional and physical responses because of past associations. Just seeing the header of an email from your ex-spouse or your boss can cause adrenaline and a sense of fear to flood your system. Seeing a picture of you and your lover on a vacation can lower your blood pressure, and for a moment you are actually back in that happy place, and you feel a flood of happy hormones wash through your system.

We are talking about intentionally creating a space with associations—good associations. Of course, intentionally creating a space for lovemaking, setting a stage with things that turn you on, and removing things that carry associations that turn you off, makes it possible to Be Here Now and have a wonderful intimate time. But it does more than that, it creates an association for the future.

Pavlov's dogs' mouths moistened at the ring of a bell. After you've had a dozen wonderful experiences in your "space," what reaction are you going to have when you see the warmth of the candlelit room, play toys at the ready, and your lover clean, shaved and smelling (and probably tasting) good? Might your heart beat a little faster? Might something else moisten at the sight? Setting the stage, intentionally creating a space for love by Turning on the Ons and Turning Off the Offs, creates a context that will over time help trigger your sexual response system.

[Michael] *Part of our "setting the stage" ritual is cleanliness, and most of the time we both shower before steamy lovemaking. Just standing there in the shower, with the candlelit room beckoning just beyond, our essential oil diffuser scenting the air and Julia waiting for me under a silken sheet, I can feel the happiness hormones wash through me, and a distinct swelling tells me that all parts of me are awakening in happy anticipation of a magical, incendiary time to come. .*

INVOLVE ALL YOUR SENSES

Why do you think we speak of sex as a sensual experience? Because it involves our senses more than our conscious minds. Sex is a physical act and therefore involves your sense of touch, but it can and should incorporate all of your other senses as well. Let's not leave the other four senses out in the cold here. In the following sections we will show you how to create a space that entrances all your senses: sight, smell, sound, touch and taste.

Sometimes when we are totally "in the groove" and are fully "Here Now," we even feel that there is a sixth sense. A sense where our bodies talk to each other in a language that is older than spoken speech. We feel what our lover is feeling, and they feel what we are feeling. Our bodies talk and know how to move together in a way that creates maximum bliss, and for a moment we merge and share something that no one outside of us will ever know. Maybe you'll find your own moment, where you will share something together with your partner no one else will ever know.

SCENTS

The sense of smell is most closely aligned with memory and emotion. More than any other sense, the mere smell of something familiar can take you back to a very specific person or time in your life. Use this to your advantage by adding smells to your environment that have positive associations for you when you are setting the stage for romance.

We have an essential oil diffuser that we turn on when we are setting our stage. We like to add several drops of lavender oil because for us that smell is connected to feelings of relaxation and peace. But the possibilities are almost limitless. You should experiment with other scents and see what combination works best for you. You can incorporate scents through the use of essential oils like we do, with scented candles or even by choosing scented soaps, lotions or massage oils.

LIGHTING

The diffuser we have in our bedroom has the added benefit of giving off a soft glow of ever-changing colored light. So, in addition to tickling our olfactory bulb, our diffuser helps create a soft romantic glow that adds to the ambience of the room as its warm light tinges the room with changing tones of red, yellow and blue.

On lighting, there is nothing like flickering candlelight or firelight. The soft, warm light shows off your skin and flowing curves without highlighting varicose veins or other imperfections you'd like to forget about right now. The flickering, moving light brings a peace similar to sitting by a river or ocean, ever changing yet ever the same.

To complement our lighting, we like to add a few well-placed candles spread about the room. The soft lighting provided by candles is a perfect way to help "turn off the off" of feeling a bit self-conscious about your aging body. Everything looks better in dim lighting! Scented candles can be another great two-for-one option—hitting both the senses of smell and sight. For our money, though, we have given up on real match-lit candles completely and made the switch to LED candles. The newer versions are almost perfect lookalikes. They flicker in a perfect simulation of candle flame and look and smell like real candles. This way romantic lighting is always just a flip of a switch away. Our candles last for years at a time and don't add any smokiness to our room. And, of course, there is no risk of setting the curtains on fire if things get extra frisky!

SOUNDS

To tickle our sense of hearing, we have experimented with lots of options. You can buy an inexpensive blue-tooth speaker that can connect to your smartphone. Once connected, you can fill the room with your favorite play list or stream some sultry music from one of the many streaming services available. A couple of caveats here. If you opt to go with a streaming channel, we cannot stress enough how important it is to pay for the premium membership so you won't have that crucial moment interrupted by an ad for hemorrhoid cream. Nothing takes you out of the moment and into your head faster than a commercial break.

Another thing we have discovered is that if we are using one of our own playlists of songs we love, this too can become distracting instead of enhancing. You don't want to have some part of your brain working away on whether the song you are hearing was originally sung by Bob Dylan or John Lennon. And you don't want to start singing along either.

The purpose of having music on during love making is to help fill the space so that you aren't feeling so self-conscious about the sounds you might be making and so that you can relax and get into the right frame of mind. We have found the best way to do this without creating unnecessary distractions is to stream a channel or playlist that features spa music, new age music or even music designed specifically to enhance a Tantric experience. What these all have in common is that there is no real melody and there are no words. They create a *feeling* but they do so without also creating something that will distract you.

If you want to get really fancy, there are apps you can download that will overlay relaxation sounds on top of the music you are streaming. Options include the sound of rain, a rushing stream or a crackling fire. These can add to the hypnotic feel of the music to help keep you present and turn off the mental chatter. One we like is called "Relax Melodies," but there are many options out there.

We have had many times where we were both really present and engaged in a sexual session and, when it was over, we suddenly become aware again that music was even on. When we are really engaged, it is almost like our ears have decided they are non-essential functions for the moment and they take a back seat to the delicious sensations our bodies are feeling.

Of course, no discussion on sensual sounds would be complete without a mention of the most erotic sound of all: the joyful moans of your partner in the throes of ecstasy. While you may have felt the need to stifle your vocalizations of pleasure in the past to ensure little ears wouldn't hear you, this is the time in your life to let them rip! It is exciting to hear the sounds and it is equally exciting to make them. Don't sensor anything. Let yourselves get truly lost in the experience.

TASTE

No discussion of a sensual banquet could be complete without the sense of taste. There are countless ways to incorporate your taste buds into your love making. Just enjoying the unique juices your partner excretes or the saltiness of his skin can be a turn-on. For more tasty fun, you can add flavored lubes and oils, or get funky with some whipped cream or chocolate sauce (put down the rubber sheets first for that one though!).

We sometimes like to create a little dessert plate to have at the ready. We will take a small bowl and line the bottom with a baggy filled with crushed ice cubes, and then place some of our favorite squares of chocolate on top to chill during our session of love making. When we are done, we can just reach over and top off the whole experience with a nip of chilled chocolate and maybe a raspberry or two.

TOUCH

When we speak of sexual pleasure, of course a huge part of that involves our sense of touch. Touch can and should involve your fingertips, but do not limit your concept of touch to just that. You can experiment with using other parts of your body, from a woman's breasts to a man's penis, to caress your lover. And of course your mouth offers a wealth of tactile pleasure options, from licking to kissing to sucking, as well as blowing warm air on your lover's skin. You can get creative with other sensations as well by adding some carefully curated props to your fun, like feathers, silky fabrics or soft furs.

One of our favorite games (see, "Putting the Play in Foreplay") involves covering one of us in a silky sheet while the other stays on top of the sheet and caresses and kisses the person below through the fabric, sometimes moving the fabric to create additional sensations and other times kissing and licking the fabric to create an almost explosive teasing sensation.

WARM AND CLEAN

Nothing turns on "the offs" more than that insecure feeling that you are not as clean as you would have liked to be now that you are having sex. For this reason, we have made it a part of our sexual ritual to shower before we meet up in bed. You can of course shower or bathe together and consider this a more active part of your foreplay, or you can each take your time alone to cleanse your body and start the transition toward romance. This is also the perfect time to attend to any grooming issues like "man-scaping," or shaving your legs. And if you use some scented soap that your partner enjoys, you can add yet another way to entice her.

For those with stiffness or joint pain, the warmth of a shower or bath can help ease these symptoms. An added plus for aging bodies.

By taking the time and effort to shower and brush your teeth before your love-making session begins, you are letting your partner know you care about them and their experience of you, and you are helping to ensure that you have one less thing to mentally obsess about when the going gets good.

And speaking of warm, let's face it. We are hoping to get naked here and we don't want to be covered in goose bumps in the process. We like to turn our heat up to about 75 degrees as we are starting to shower so that the room will be nice and toasty for us when we are ready to be together. Even if you like making love under the blankets, a cold draft that blows in when one of you moves is going to ruin your "Be Here Now" moment. Turning up the heat for an hour or two every now and then is not going to destroy the planet, and it just might ignite your love life.

DÉCOR

Another thing to consider is the vibe of the room where you will be making love. Is the floor covered with dirty laundry? Are the dressers or tables covered with piles of papers? Are the sheets clean and silky and inviting? Remember our goal is to help you Be Here Now. If your room is littered with things that will remind you of the countless other things you need to be doing, you are going to be hitting the brakes on your sexual response system. Take that extra time to make the space warm and inviting and be sure it does not trigger any work or chore stress for you.

If you are planning to make love in your bedroom, you might want to take a little time to think about the kinds of associations you have with that room. Has this always been a sanctuary for the two of you? A place of peace and saucy sex? Or is it an uncomfortable reminder of all the sex you have not been having—that damned bed serving as the elephant in the room? Is this where you tend to have your arguments?

If your associations with your bedroom are less than positive, it is worth thinking about how to address that piece. One option would be to try to consecrate the space in a new way. Is there some sort of ritual you can create that will change the space emotionally for you? This might involve literally cleaning it up or changing the décor to signal a fresh start, or it might be something more symbolic like burning some sage to clear out the negative vibes or hanging a piece of art or putting a sign on the door to rededicate the space to one of love.

If you don't feel you can adequately address the history of negative energy in the room, it may make sense to come up with a plan for a Fresh Start space. Now that the kids are likely gone chances are good that you have another bedroom or two at your disposal in your living space. Why not adopt one of these rooms as your own special place for loving. Again, you might wish to change the bedding so that it feels new and inviting to you and you might choose to decorate it with photos or other mementos that remind you of the happiest times you have shared together. Treat this space as a sacred spot for your renewed love making adventure. Use it only for those good times.

READY AND WAITING

"Hey, where did we put the lube? Did we clean the sex toys after the last time? Did we charge them up? Wow, I'm thirsty, but too lazy to go downstairs and get a glass of water."

Don't let this happen to you. Anything that causes you to uncouple and reach into your nightstand drawers, trying to find something by touch in a darkened room is sure to take you out of the moment. Have it all ready, waiting, and within easy reach. As you are racing your engine up a mountain of passion toward a mind-blowing climax, going faster and faster, the last thing you need is to take a time out to stop and check the oil.

Would a drink of ice water taste good after a hot session, or maybe as a little break between bouts? Have it ready. If you use sex toys, have them clean, charged and waiting within easy reach. If you want chocolate afterwards, have it chilling on ice.

We love using lube, and use at least a little in most sessions. And we like it hot. There is nothing like having hot oil dripped on your aroused body, and having your lover smooth it out over you with his hands and body. We used to try warming the oil in hot water in the sink, or even in a big bowl of hot water sitting by the bed.

Ready and Waiting

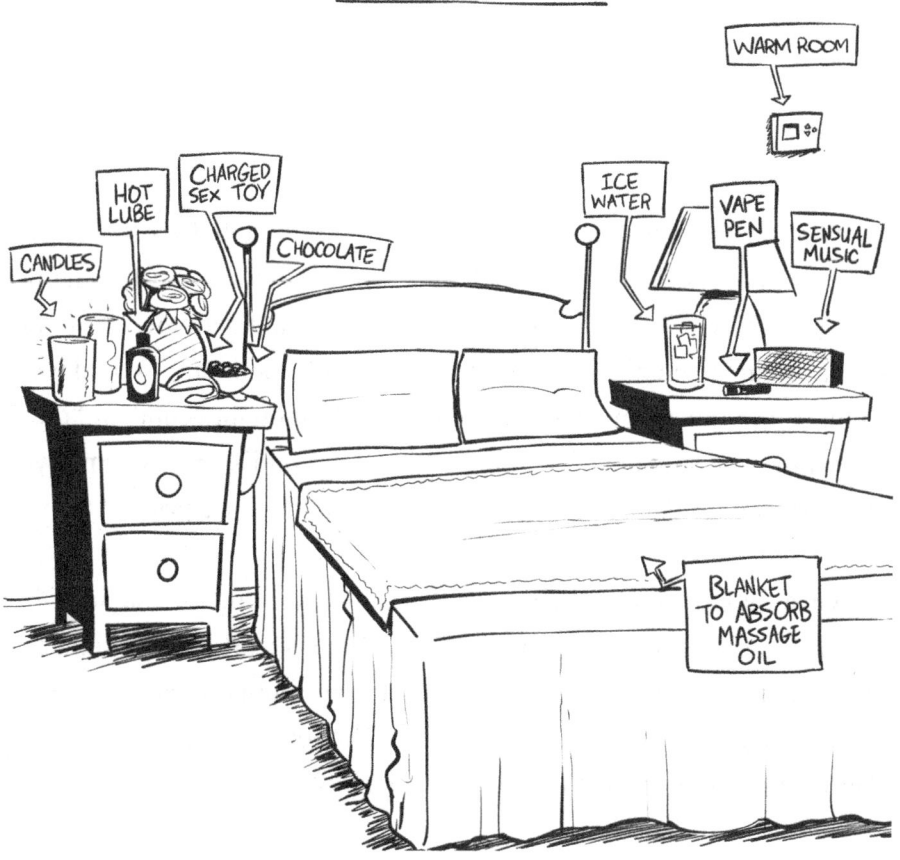

This was good, but the water soon cooled and the extra water dripping onto the sheets was a turn-off. Then we found the perfect solution. We have a little personal heating pad that we wrap tightly around the bottle of lube. We use some of the cord slack to wrap around our little package to keep things snug and then plug the heating pad in and turn it on. We put the heating-pad-wrapped lube into the top nightstand drawer, opened just enough to easily grab the bottle when needed. Hot, sensual oil at the ready.

WHAT DO I CALL IT?

Speaking of "Offs," a single wrong word can cool passion as fast as dropping a hot iron into an ice bath. Yes, we are speaking of how you talk about you and your partner's genitalia.

What is common about all these names: cunt, snatch, fuck hole, poon, twat, pussy, cock, dick, junk, prick? Each of these common slang names for penis and vagina are also all terms of abuse and derision. How you speak about something affects how you feel about it. Would your feelings for your lover change if you mentally thought "cunt" or "dick" every time you saw them? Would it help your child's self-esteem if you nicknamed your daughter "twat," or your son "the little prick"?

We are talking about the mystical organs that bring the magic of life into the world, and the only parts of your body specifically designed to give you steamy, incendiary, mind-shattering mutual pleasure. Your genitalia should be revered, treasured, and honored, rather than derided. Can't we do better than cunt, pussy, and dick?

You will notice that we have generally used the very generic words "penis" and "vagina" to describe our beautiful and magical organs, but that's not what we say to each other while making love. There are people who get turned on using "dirty" language, who may be wired to get excited by doing something sinful or taboo and use derisive or taboo language to describe their sexual organs. Hey, if it works for you, great. But many people—particularly women—will feel better about their own bodies if they know their lover respects and worships that part of them.

Somehow in western society in the last century we have gotten off course. It is only lately that the common words used to describe genitalia are almost all abusive. Here are some common phrases out of the past, and the year they first appeared.

For Her:

- The Altar of Venus (1584)
- Phoenix's nest (1618)
- Nature's treasury (1635)
- Mount Pleasant (1748)
- Petticoat Lane (1790)
- Cyprian fountain (1846)

For Him:

- Maypole (1621)
- Master John Goodfellow (1653)
- Gentleman Usher (1719)
- Silent flute (1720)
- Arbor vitae (1732)
- Impudence (1783)
- Cyprian scepter (1653)
- Don Cypriano (1653)

We're not sure where all these references to Cyprus come from. Was it a spicy place it the 1600s? It makes us want to visit there and find out!

Many non-Western cultures are also not burdened with derisive or abusive terms for man and lady bits. In Hindu and Tantric society, they say *Yoni*, which means "divine passage" or "place of origin," to refer to the vagina, and *Lingam* and *Vajra* for penis. In Chinese society, you may say "lotus," "thousand-petaled lotus flower," "pearly gate," "jade gate" or "jade garden" for vagina, and "jade stalk" or "wand of light" for penis.

Many women internally cringe every time they hear their lover say one of the more derisive slang terms, even if they've been hearing them for decades. Sure, you may feel silly speaking of your "wand of light" or her "jade garden," but, well first, lighten up! Secondly, ask your partner what terms they would like you to use, or use a poetic or romantic term spontaneously, and you may see instant benefits. Be inventive, romantic, erotic, and kind (see our section on "Kindness"). Here are a few terms to help start your imagination:

For Her –
- Pink Pearl
- Flower
- Her core
- Her center
- Her sex
- Her essence
- Pool of moisture
- Mons
- Sugar walls
- Fragrant curls
- Honeypot
- Jade Garden

For Him -
- Manhood
- His sex
- Love muscle
- Magic wand
- Mount Vesuvius
- Staff
- Rod
- Shaft
- Love missle
- Wand of light
- Stalk
- Joystick
- Wand of Light

Or just make up your own pet name. It doesn't matter if it might sound silly to other people, especially people who wish they were having the kind of wonderful sex you are (or soon will be) having. This is an intimate thing between the two of you. It's not like you are going to post it on Facebook.

Sticks and Stones May Break My Bones But Words Will *Always* Hurt Me.

[Julia] *When I hear words like "puss,y" "snatch" or "cunt," I can literally feel my body shutting down. There is an inward contraction happening, like some steel door snapping shut. In contrast, when my lover refers to my jade garden (my poetic term of choice), the exact opposite happens. I feel a warm sensation radiate through me, and an opening, as if my heart and body are expanding. These are genuine physical sensations based on my emotional response to the words used. Words matter. Use them wisely.*

BREATHING

We spoke above about how to set the mood physically, but without doubt, the most important aspect of setting the mood is being present mentally. This has been our greatest challenge over the years as we have navigated our way through life's twists and turns—issues with kids, jobs, ex-spouses, and every little thing in between. All of these are sex drive crushers. So how can we stop the mental clutter from overtaking us when we want to connect with our partner?

The two best tricks we have discovered are some breathing exercises and the judicious use of legal pot. While you can literally just spoon one another and take a few deep breaths, we have some more detailed breathing exercises below that you might consider trying. (See "Tantra for Fun" under the chapter on "Mating Rituals.") It is amazing how this simple act can effectively sweep out the cobwebs of the day and bring you to a place of peace. Inhale, hold, exhale. After several breaths, swap who is spooning whom. Breath into your partner's warm neck. Feel your bodies rising and falling with each breath. You focus on breathing and how your lover's body feels against you, and the world begins to recede.

While we have had incredible success by breathing together, we know that there are those times where it is just not sufficient to take away the stress of the day. Adding the occasional hit of legal cannabis to the start of our love-making sessions has been nothing short of revolutionary for us. You can read much more about this in our sections under "Sex and Cannabis" above and "The Cannabis Ritual" below. We are quite honestly astounded at how effective a small amount of pot can be at stopping the spinning mind, shutting everything external down and just helping us feel focused and present. It also helps tune down any inhibitions, so we come to our session feeling more open and ready to connect.

THE CANNABIS RITUAL

So, you and your lover are warm and clean. Hot oil, toys, water and chocolate are all within easy reach. Luscious scents, flickering candlelight and softly playing erotic music turn the room into a magical lair where the world can recede and you can live moment to moment. What now?

There are no rules. With the stage set, maybe you won't need games like those found in our "Mating Rituals" section below to build your arousal. Perhaps a few breathing exercises or a round of "Tantra for Fun" will take the rest of the world away. But sometimes the world just won't let you alone, and no matter how much you want to, you just can't "Be Here Now." Thoughts of the argument you had at work, the needed plumbing repair, or the dinner party you need to plan for just keep intruding. No matter how skillfully and lovingly your partner touches you, the psychic baggage from the day just won't let you be.

Don't waste the night. This is where a tiny bit of cannabis—often just a single toke—can help immensely. Read all of our sections in "Sex and Cannabis." Share a disposable vape stick or enjoy a few hits of flower with your lover, and just let the world go. You will start to feel the change within seconds, and the full change within 5 minutes. If you still hear the world shouting at you, take another hit. Remember, the effect will vary from person to person and even night to night, and if this is your first time, there's a good chance you won't feel anything. But if it works, it can be truly magical. You may even feel freer with your body than you ever have. Your anxieties may melt away along with the psychic baggage of the day.

Make your own ritual. No rules. You could have some cannabis and take a bath together, or dance together, your clothes disappearing as the dance goes on. Maybe with a single toke you are already there, in your lover's arms savoring their touch. The outside world has disappeared, and you are beginning those timeless moments that make life worth living.

Do you need pot to have great sex? Absolutely not. It's not about the pot but about getting into the loving state of mind, and we have described many ways to help you do this. But if you have done everything you can to turn off the offs and turn on the ons, and the world still won't leave you alone, you may find this is one way to turn a potentially frustrating evening into an evening of sweet sensuality worth remembering. You may find yourselves laying back as we have many times, spent and warmly slick from sweat and oils, and saying with a smile, "Now THAT's incendiary sex."

MATING RITUALS

Putting the "Play" back into "Foreplay"

The candles are flickering, music is softly playing, and you are both warm, clean and naked. Maybe you've done a few breathing exercises and had a toke of pot. The cares of the day have mostly swirled away. You are living moment to moment, and your mind is on your partner and the sensations of your partner's skin against yours. Congratulations, you are in a "Be Here Now" moment.

What now? Just getting to "Be Here Now" is a huge step, and you could have foreplay and sex as you've done it countless times before, and without the swirl of worries in your head, that can be wonderful. However, there is more. We want to show you a few games to put the "Play" back into "Foreplay." Games that create sexual tension, building up the erotic energy to the point that the dam breaks and washes you in a flood of orgasmic bliss. Games that explore sensual delights you may never have experienced, or that stretch your lovemaking into new sexual areas to explore.

Here we detail some of our favorite games. Experiment with some of these or try to come up with some of your own. The point is to have fun, but also to provide a little bit of structure and focus so that you are not as likely to get trapped in a destructive head space or feel like you are falling back into a stale routine. Even in a "Be Here Now" setting, your regular sex routine may be so well known to you that thoughts of the day might intrude, or there may be a bit of boredom with the "same old, same old." And as the famous Dr. Ruth says, "Boredom is a lot more dangerous to a relationship than any other factor."

"Tantra for Fun" is the only game where you have to remember anything, and that's only the order in which to pleasure your Chakra's (the mnemonic "Heart and Soul, and Bottom's Up" is all you'll need). Even on days when we're tired and stressed, "Tanta for Fun" has rarely failed to engage our senses and build sexual energy.

"Guided Erotic Massage" can become addicting. At once both ultimately relaxing and sensuously stimulating. Some say that the key to a happy and fulfilled life is to find your comfort zone—and then leave it. The best things often happen outside your comfort zone. Many of our Mating Rituals such as "Better to Give or Receive? Try Both!" "Covered but Accessible," "Hot and Cold," and "Blindfolds" will push you into new areas of sensual delight, where you may find erotic joys that you haven't dreamed of. "Sexy Reading"and "Talk Clean to Me" will engage your creativity and imagination and help re-enliven a sexual fantasy life that may have withered over the years.

> **Some say that the key to a happy and fulfilled life is to find your comfort zone—and then leave it. The best things often happen outside your comfort zone.**

Take our Mating Rituals as springboards in which to launch your own games and rituals. Don't take any of these games too seriously. Adapt ours and invent and create your own. If a game doesn't end up working for you, laugh together about it and strike it off your list. If you get so hot that you can't finish a game and end up having insanely steamy mind-blowing sex, don't worry. Unlike most games, these are the kind where you can win without even finishing.

TANTRA FOR FUN

We know not everyone is lucky enough (yet) to live in a state where recreational pot is legal and easily accessible so fear not—we have many great options for helping you get present and "Be Here Now" with your lover, with or without pot. "Tantra for Fun" is a breathing exercise, but with an erotic twist. Breathing together is one of the best ways to get present with your lover. Take the time to slow down and breath together. This may sound glib but trust us, it really works. Just lying next to one another and taking a series of slow, deep breaths can help get you present and relaxed, but we are going to show you how to turn breathing into a sensual symphony.

You may feel that Tantric Sex is just too far out there for you. "I don't even own love beads," you might say, "No way can I get into a lotus position," or "Is this where I breath out of my left eye while you're breathing out of your right eye, or is it the other way around?"

Don't worry. This is fun and easy, and if it hadn't lead us into many nights and afternoons of steamy, incendiary sex, it wouldn't be in our book. This is our own wild adaptation of the "Nurturing Meditation" that we originally found in the classic guide, "Tantra, the Art of Conscious Loving," by Charles and Caroline Muir. And it all starts with Chakras.

Chakras are a series of energy centers in the body believed to control and contain the psychic energy through which one may achieve physical ecstasy and spiritual unity in many Eastern cultures. Now we know, this all sounds pretty Woo-Woo, but we promise you don't have to study ancient texts or stare deeply into each other eyes for ten hours without moving in order to reap some benefit here. Just stay with us and trust the process. You will need to take a few moments to learn the location of the seven Chakras in order to do this properly. To help, we are including a diagram below.

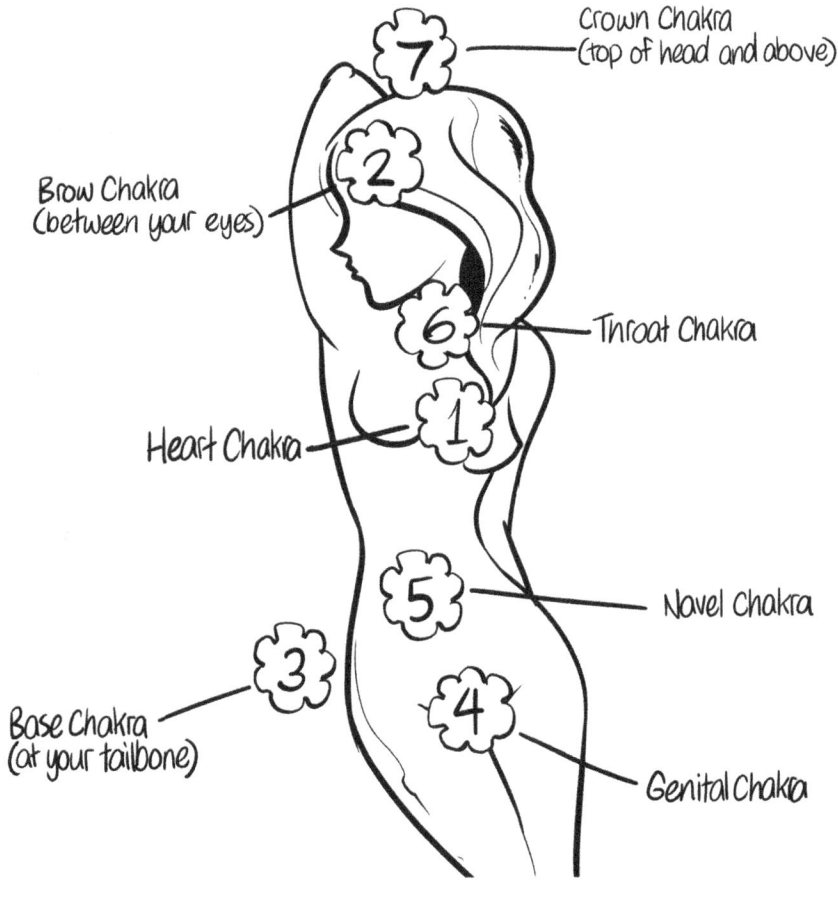

The Chakras start at the base of your spine and work their way up to (and through) the top of your head. Like your spine, they essentially form a column that goes through the center of your body, but instead of being made of bones and nerves, the column is an energetic one. We like to visualize a column of light.

In each of the breathing exercises below, you will be concentrating on, touching, massaging, breathing on, kissing and/or licking your partner's Chakras in the order as numbered in the diagram. Take a few minutes getting this part down so that you can stay present and focused as you are executing it. Here is the order you want to focus on:

1. Heart Chakra. The Heart Chakra is the center of love, compassion, harmony and peace. We fall in love through our heart Chakra.

2. Third Eye or Brow Chakra. This is the third eye, and since the eyes are the windows to our soul you can think of this as the Soul Chakra. This Chakra is concerned with inner vision, intuition and wisdom.

3. Base Chakra. Think of this as being at the base of your spine, near your tailbone. It is the only Chakra that you should visualize as being on the back of your body. The others all run up the front of your body. This is the Chakra that is concerned with earthly grounding and physical survival.

4. Genitals Chakra. We just call this the "genitals Chakra" but you might want to come up with something more poetic to refer to. This Chakra is concerned with desire, pleasure, sexuality, and creativity. Sorry, you still can't linger more than three breaths here.

5. Navel Chakra. The Naval Chakra is located around and above the navel, and is the seat of your emotional life, with feelings of personal power, laughter, joy and anger.

6. Throat Chakra. This is the Chakra of communication, creativity, self-expression and judgement. It is concerned with healing, transformation and purification.

7. Crown Chakra. Located at the top of your head, it is concerned with understanding, acceptance and bliss, and is said to be your personal pathway to God, and to your Divine purpose and personal destiny.

An easy mnemonic device for this is to think, "Heart and Soul," and then "Bottom's Up." In other words, you will start at the heart Chakra. Next comes the brow Chakra, the window to your soul. From there, it's Bottom's Up--you start at the base Chakra and work your way up to the top, the Crown Chakra, skipping the two Chakras you already did at the beginning.

In their book, the Muirs use the analogy of strings of a guitar. Each string vibrates at its own frequency and gives off a different tone. When they are all in tune, the strings create harmony. Your goal is to tune your energy centers so that they are humming along in alignment with your partner's. Again, stay with us. We know this all sounds pretty out there.

We call this a breathing exercise but we really think it is more helpful to think of this as a game. The term "exercise" makes it sound like a chore, and believe us, this is not a chore.

Chakra breathing is one of our favorite ways to start off a romance session, especially if one or both of us are feeling a bit distracted from the emotional clutter of the day. We can't think of a time when this failed to bring us to the present—ready, willing and able.

There are three levels of this game: *Slow and Steady* (concentrate only on your Chakras, no touching), *Kick it Up a Notch* (touching and massaging Chakras allowed), and *Oh My God!* (breathing on, kissing, licking your lover's Chakras). Here's how they work:

Level One: Slow and Steady

Here you want to spoon with your lover, with both of you lying on your left side (this is for reasons of energy flow according to Tantric texts). If one of you is feeling less grounded or more needy as you start this, that person should assume the inside position, with the other partner taking the more nurturing role. You can also go through this a couple of times, switching positions between sets. It may take two or three rounds through the series to really achieve that feeling of peace and presence.

You want to both be comfortable here. If you are the person on the outside, you might slip your bottom arm under your partner's neck or pillow, and place your top hand on your partner's chest, belly or genitals. You want to feel connected and cozy.

You are going to be doing a series of slow deep breaths, breathing together at the same time and pace. There are four steps to each breath: You will inhale deeply, hold it a beat, exhale slowly, and hold another beat before you start again with the inhalation. With each set of three breaths (inhale, hold, exhale, hold—for three sets), you will focus on a different Chakra in your mind. Although it sounds pretty out there, the mental focus is an important part of this game. We like to imagine a pinwheel at each Chakra space, and when we are focusing on a given Chakra, we try to make it spin in our minds.

We like to have the person in the nurturing position (the one on the outside) quietly signal the order to their partner to be sure you are both acting in harmony. In other words, take a moment to just synchronize your breathing and then when you are ready, have the Nurturer quietly whisper "Heart Chakra." After three breaths, he will whisper "Brow Chakra," and so on. We cannot tell you how many times we have started this when we were thinking, "There is no way this is going to work for me today since I am feeling too ___ (fill in the blank)." But damn if it hasn't worked every single time. That is not to say that every time we have done this we have gone on to have incendiary sex. But we can say that this has worked every time to get us settled, present, relaxed and ready to try.

We can't explain how or why it works. We just know it does. Try it. Get outside your comfort zone. We are guessing that your comfort zone has sort of worn out its welcome lately anyway or you probably wouldn't be reading this book. You literally have nothing to lose but a few minutes of your time, and you just might be surprised by what you will gain.

Level Two: Kick it Up A Notch

With Level Two, you will do the same thing you did in Level One, but instead of the Nurturer just verbally narrating the Chakra order, he will also use his hands. When we are playing at this level, the Nurturing partner will touch the body part most closely associated with the Chakra we are focusing on. We have found it can be really helpful to move your hand in a clockwise circular motion over the spot in question to simulate a spinning motion instead of just holding steady, so that you are reminding your partner to get their Chakra spinning. (Remember the pinwheel image.)

This really starts to get the sexual energy moving. You will notice that certain Chakras feel more charged to you than others. For Julia, the base Chakra provides a surprising amount of sexual energetic flow.

Again, you can go through this series multiple times, switching spooning positions if you desire.

Level Three: Oh My God!

Once you have gotten comfortable with the basic series (at Level One and/or Level Two), you can start to move into a more sexually charged level of play by running through the series one more time at Level Three. (Or two or three or four more times... Trust us, this level rocks!)

For this version, the Nurturing Partner is no longer spooning the other partner but instead will be moving herself around her partner's Chakras, literally breathing into them. The receiving partner will lie on his back and the Nurturing Partner will start by placing her mouth over his heart Chakra, using a combination of warm breath, hand pressure, and licks and kisses (get creative here) on and around the Chakra to stimulate the Chakra in play. After three breaths at the heart, the Nurturer will move to the brow. This may involve the Nurturer straddling her partner, pretty much genitals to genitals so that she can position her lips on her lover's forehead and breathe, kiss, lick, etc. this space.

After working on the brow Chakra it is "Bottom's Up" time so the Nurturer will turn her partner over so she can access his back, working her magic on his base Chakra. After this Chakra, she will turn him back over onto his back to hit the genitals, navel, throat and crown Chakras, again, moving over her partner as needed, sometimes straddling him or otherwise caressing him with her body as she goes. You can get very creative here when it comes to the genitals Chakra, licking, sucking, and blowing your warm breath in a way that will really start to get the sexual energy flowing. Remember, just three breathes each. This can be a delicious tease since the time spent here will be limited, so you will get your lover yearning for more as you move on to the next Chakra.

This game will not only help you get relaxed and present, but will likely leave you begging for more. Many is the time we started on this journey and didn't end up finishing it because we literally couldn't take it anymore and just had to have each other. Don't take this too seriously. If you're ready to go straight for "Kick it Up a Notch" or "Oh My God!," do it. Just keep the erotic tension building by trying to keep to the three breaths each, at least until you truly can't help yourself. We hope you will find the same sort of ecstatic response to this game that we have.

GUIDED EROTIC MASSAGE

Massage and sex go together like red wine and chocolate. If you are stressed out and your muscles are tense, blood flow to your genitalia will be compromised, making sexual arousal nearly impossible. To combat this issue, we highly recommend you incorporate some erotic massage into your romance repertoire. A good sexual experience cannot happen unless you wake up your sexual energy and allow it to both flow and build.

However, having a massage manual open on one side of the bed, and stopping intermittently to read a set of instructions is not going to make for the hottest of massages. Anything that takes you out of the moment and keeps you from "Being Here Now" is a turn off to your erotic energy, and stopping to read an instruction manual is definitely an "off."

Unless you are highly experienced at giving erotic massages, even trying to memorize a series of massage techniques is distracting for the massage giver, as you focus mentally on the list of techniques in your head instead of focusing on the touch, taste and scent of your partner. Your partner will feel consciously or unconsciously that you are in your own head, and not totally "Here."

The answer is an auditory guided massage. An audio track that smoothly takes you from one massage technique to another, without the distraction of reading or remembering. A guided massage, so long as it's slow and smooth, allows you to "Be Here Now," and just enjoy and revel in the sensations.

We originally thought that this chapter would be very short. Several years ago we found a wonderful video by acclaimed sexologist Jaiya (yes, like Cher and Madonna, it is apparently just Jaiya), who had created a guided massage video called "Erogenous Zones and Orgasmic Massage" as part of her "Red Hot Touch" video series.

We had intended to describe how guided erotic massage could be used in your love play, and to point you to this great video. However, sadly the video is apparently no longer available (and no, you can't borrow our copy). We then scoured the internet looking for similar guided massages, and unfortunately everything we found was terrible.

Guided massages have been for us a wonderful way to build erotic energy, and have been part of some of our best sensual experiences. We didn't want you to miss the opportunity to enjoy this, so we decided if you can't find it, make it!

While the sensual but tasteful video portion of Jaiya's video is instructive, we found that it is not really necessary, and that an audio guided massage is totally adequate. To that end, we made and used our own guided massage audio, and the script to this is found at the end of this book. For us it was even better than Jaiya at building our erotic energy. After all, we made it to our own sexual tastes! You can create your own audio guided massage, using the script found near the back of this book in "Appendix: Erotic Guided Massage Script" or by adapting it to your own particular pleasures. Simply read the script, slowly and sexily and with the appropriate pauses, into a recording device like your smartphone and then play it back for both of you via a blue tooth speaker and enjoy an erotic massage experience. The script we have written will result in an approximately 40-45 minute massage, but of course you can adapt it to be longer or shorter to your pleasure.

Creating your own guided erotic massage will take some effort, but isn't that a great gift to give your lover, letting them know how much you care about their pleasure? You may find, as we did, that just making the guided massage and imagining it as you go is a stimulating experience and a bit of foreplay on its own. We hope you also find that actually doing your own erotic massage leads to some incredible, incendiary sex, just as we did.

One final note on this topic. We know that as we age, our stamina and hand strength can diminish, and for those with arthritis in their hands this may be especially true. Don't feel like you have to commit to a long full-body session. Even mini five-minute sessions can provide tremendous comfort and pleasure. One area to focus on is the buttocks and upper thighs. We all carry a lot of tension in these areas and helping to ease this will greatly increase blood flow to the genital region, thus allowing for more sexual arousal. One great tip we learned from Jaiya is that the gluteal fold (the crease under your butt cheeks) is actually quite a powerful erogenous zone. Spend some time rubbing and pressing along that area on your partner's body. You may be surprised by the results!

BETTER TO GIVE OR RECEIVE? TRY BOTH!

In many relationships one partner tends to be the passive one, and one partner the active one during lovemaking. If this describes your relationship, then you may be missing a world of erotic pleasures. People who have played the active role their entire lives often find a joy they never knew in being passive and accepting love and touch. People who have always been comfortable being passive can find a new confidence and a thrill that will translate to sexual energy by being the active creator of their partner's pleasure.

Here each partner takes turns being the giver or the receiver, where one of you will be the giver and the other one the receiver for a set period of time. We like to put on some music and use the song length as our timer, swapping roles at the end of each song. You could also set a timer for somewhere between three and five minutes if you would prefer to do this without a sound track. The rules are straight forward.

The receiver lies back in a "ready, willing and able" position while the giver attends to her body in any way he feels inspired to do—touching, licking, kissing, sucking. Don't just hit the usual suspects here. Move around your lover's body and try to discover secret pleasure zones. You could start by sucking your lover's toes, or by lightly stroking the insides of her elbows. The only real rule is that the receiver must passively receive—they cannot also be touching or stimulating their partner. This is meant to build sexual tension, so you may want to work your way up to and near your lover's genitals, but don't spend too much time there just yet. You pleasure your partner for the full length of a song (or until your timer goes off), and when that song is over, you switch roles. No matter how good things were getting, you have to force yourselves to stop and switch. Enjoy the back and forth for a couple of rounds, perhaps getting increasingly more genital-focused as you go.

You could experiment with having the receiver wear a blind fold or sleep mask so that they won't be able to anticipate what is coming next. Particularly if you are used to being the receiver, blindfold your partner when the times comes for you to be the active one. For many people (especially women), this will release their inhibitions and allow them to do things they never considered before— things that will have their lover squirming with the need to touch them and have them, heightened by the requirement to lay and just take the sensual delights you are providing.

You can give this game an extra tension-builder by imposing the rule of EBG: Everything But the Genitals. Feel free to come as close as you can to your partner's genitals to build that anticipation, but do not actually stimulate them, except perhaps with your hot breath, or by lightly brushing your hair across their most sensitive spots.

This EBG version of Give and Receive can be particularly helpful as a stand-alone experience for couples trying to rebuild after a long sexual drought. By taking genital stimulation off the table, both partners can relax into the experience of tactile reconnection without the fear that their lover is expecting this to lead to sex. As we discuss in our section "When It's Been a Loooong Time," affirmatively removing sex from the agenda for the evening will help both partners enjoy their experience of physical connection without the fear that if they get into the experience they might be sending a signal to their lover that they want more than they are ready to provide.

BODY MAPPING

Here again, you take turns playing giver or receiver, but in this game you will want to give yourselves a more luxurious amount of time to explore. The idea is to explore your lover's body like a cartographer, but instead of trying to capture their physical shape, you are trying to map out their sensory hot spots. You may want to do this a bit systematically, starting either at the top or bottom of the body and working your way to the other end. And of course there is both the front and back side of the body to explore. You can decide if you want to try to cover the whole body one at a time, or take turns mapping smaller portions.

Try different types of caresses, as well as kissing and tongue play to experiment with what sorts of sensations bring excitement to your lover. This is a good game to start with the EBG (Everything But Genitals) version. After all, we are trying like explorers to find the secret springs of erotic pleasures, and we already know about the genitals! There are a welter of erogenous zones that can be found with a little loving exploration. Lick, caress and kiss under the chin, the back of the knees, and the underside of the arms. Massage the scalp, the temples and the little divots in the back of the neck where the skull meets the neck. Take a handful of hair and pull gently. Squeeze the earlobes and gently pull on them. Find the pleasure points at the center of the palms and feet. Suck on toes and fingertips.

We say "start" with EBG, but of course a thorough mapping of the genitals may also lead to little spots of stimulation you never knew you had. Particularly for women, the system of nerves that can be stimulated toward orgasm extends throughout the lower torso. Touches and licks to the inner thigh, rubbing the muscles just above the pubis, and stroking the anus, the crease of the ass, and the perineum (the space between anus and vagina), can all stimulate the network of nerves that increases sexual energy. Pressing your thumbs and massaging into the gluteal fold, the crease where the buttocks meets the legs, is a little-known but very effective erogenous zone. Also, massaging some of the little divots in the muscles of the buttocks can feel wonderful, as well as points alongside the tailbone.

Don't rush. Exploring and making love very, very, slowly builds intimacy, and keeps your partner from being startled when you rush to a new and intimate spot that they've never had touched or kissed before. Good communication here is ideal, but even if you are not comfortable expressing yourself verbally, your lover can try to tune in to your subtle body language, the sighs, moans and squiggles of delight should help clue him in to your pleasure.

And this game is for the explorer as well. Revel in the different scents and tastes of your partner. Explore the different textures, the luscious wet smoothness of the inner labia, the softness of the space between the toes, the little ledge under the head of the penis, the roughness of the G-spot when your partner is excited.

When you've found a spot that delights and excites your partner, don't forget about it! Bring it into your lovemaking. There is gold hidden in those hills and valleys. Go out like the explorers of old, and bring home the treasure.

COVERED BUT ACCESIBLE

In all of lovemaking there is a special tension, a building of arousal and erotic energy, by being almost, but not quite, there. When you feel your partner's breath on your sensitive spots, knowing her lips are just millimeters away. When your partner slides his hands softly down almost to your genitals, but not quite, resting so close you can feel the tiny distance between you.

A great way of creating that sexual tension—and keeping an arousal building millimeter between you—just requires a silky, smooth sheet. Take that silky sheet and place it over your lover, while you remain on top of it. All of your caressing, kissing, and licking will be done with you on top of the sheet while your partner is underneath it. You can even use the sheet as a tool to caress your partner by slowly moving the fabric across her body in sensual ways.

The sheet performs several functions here. First, it is a physical barrier between you and your lover so there is literally no way you can engage in intercourse with the sheet there. This hard-line boundary helps to build the sexual tension. And second, it adds a sensual element to your play because everything feels a little different than what you are used to feeling when you are in bed with your partner. Notice the way the sheet caresses your skin. Can you feel the moisture of his kisses through the fabric? How about the warmth of her breath? It is just another way to change things up so that the experience feels fresh and exciting, all of which helps you to stay present with what is happening right now.

The feeling of the sliding, silky sheet itself can be so erotic that some women and even a few men can orgasm without skin touching skin. You can feel the heat of your partner's breath through the sheet and even perhaps the moisture from their mouth or vagina. Plus, you may find that the feeling of actual skin against skin after denying yourself during the game may be a new peak of erotic sensation.

If you and your partner are trying to ease yourselves back into a sexual relationship after a long hiatus (See "When it's Been a Loooong Time"), this is a great way to play together that is relatively non-threatening. Under these circumstances, you want to take away the pressure that one of you expects to have intercourse so that the more reluctant partner can relax into the moment and feel safe doing so. The sheet helps solidify that you mean business here. It is not physically possible to have sex while playing this game, but it is possible to have fun.

HOT AND COLD

As you've probably picked up by now, we love a good hot oil massage. The delicious feeling of the almost-too-hot oil dribbling onto your skin, to be quickly smoothed over by your lover's hands and body is not a feeling you want to miss. It awakens the skin and the senses and focuses your thoughts on sensations alone.

On a hot and steamy night you can take those sensations even farther, and awaken your skin to lovely extremes that can release a torrent of sexual energy. Imagine for a moment that you are laying on your back, blindfolded, with your body alive and literally rising up to meet the drips of hot oil hitting your skin. Suddenly, something cold as ice traces up your stomach and across your breasts and makes you gasp. The cold feels intense, not cold, but like a different kind of heat. Your senses reel. But then, you feel the furnace heat of your partners hot lips and tongue as your icy-hot chest is bathed in a delicious wet heat, ending with his lips, cool from warming your body, kissing yours.

That's what we mean by hot and cold. In this game, you are again trying to tickle your senses with some new experiences, this time with the extremes of hot and cold. You might have fun using a blindfold on your partner so that he won't be able to anticipate what is coming next. The surprise element is yet another way to help you both stay present with the experience.

For the erotic chill, you might try things like ice cubes (real or fake ice cubes) or a chilled wash cloth. We have experimented with freezing little teething toys that we purchased just for this purpose in the baby aisle of the grocery store. This turned out to be a fun way to get that delicious chill feeling without the watery mess that comes with melted ice or wet wash cloths, and with the added benefit of yet more textures to play with. Many of these toys are soft, rubbery and nubby, all of which can feel interesting when used to caress your lover. And for an added bonus—all those fun colors and shapes! Plus, think of how prepared you will seem when the grandbaby comes over to visit and has a tooth ache! For best results, place the teething toys in the freezer for at least 30 minutes before your romance session begins.

For exploring the hot side of things, nothing beats the feel of warm massage oil or lube. (See our section on choosing the right lube.) We used to heat our oil by soaking the bottle in warm water first. We tried doing this in the bathroom sink, and also tried doing this in a bowl that we placed at the bedside. Both of these worked sufficiently well to heat the oil, but we always ended up dripping water on the sheets. Our new life hack to solve this problem is to heat the oil with the help of a personal heating pad. We plug the pad into an outlet near the bed and then roll the pad around the bottle of lube snugly. We then wrap some of the cord around our little "bundle of joy" a few times to keep the pad tightly in place around the bottle. All of this is strategically placed at arm's reach inside the top bedside table drawer, opened just enough to access it when needed.

(Here's a note on what NOT to do to heat up your lube: do not attempt to heat it in a pan on the stove. We tried this once with our silicone lube and it was virtually impossible to get that oily film off the pan.)

You can get creative here about what you will do with your hot and cold items, and whether you will be taking turns or playing at the same time. The point, again, is to kick your sensual perceptions up a notch and to be surprised by the variety of ways you can feel.

SEXY READING

When we first got together one of the things we discovered we had in common was a mutual love of Jane Austen and her novel, "Pride and Prejudice." (OK, if we are being honest here, it was Julia's love for the novel and Michael's love for the BBC adaptation of it. We both agreed the American version with Keira Knightley was too abridged.) For our first Valentine's Day together, Michael bought a novel by the contemporary author Linda Berdoll, whose book "Mr. Darcy Takes a Wife" (with a bit of emphasis on the "Takes"), picks up the story of Elizabeth and Darcy pretty much where Jane Austen had left off in her book.

The author was no longer constrained by the morals of Jane Austen's time, however, so the book was quite a bit saucier than the original. In this updated version, our favorite couple were quite randy and could barely keep their hands off each other. Ms. Berdoll continued Darcy and Lizzie's erotic exploits in "Darcy & Elizabeth," "The Ruling Passion," and "The Darcys: New Pleasures." I can't say that these books are going to win any Pulitzer prizes, but it was a fun read and definitely fit into the category of erotica, helping to get our juices flowing.

We created a little ritual of climbing into bed together and taking turns reading the novel aloud. You may not be able to recall the feeling you had as a child when you were tucked snuggly into bed and your parent read a bedtime story to you, but perhaps you can conjure up that image of reading with a child of your own. There are few things in life that are as relaxing as being read to in the warmth and comfort of your bed. While those child-related images are sweet and chaste, being read to by your lover can be a very different but equally relaxing kind of experience.

We have found this to be a great form of foreplay on a number of fronts. First, it helps achieve that "Be Here Now" goal of getting you super relaxed and present. Having to focus on a story helps divert your brain from those other vexing thoughts such as the problem you had at work that day or the deadline you are not sure you will be able to meet tomorrow. Second, it helps you connect with your partner because you will (ideally) be naked together in bed, snuggled up to one another. In addition to this physical connection, you are jointly focused on the same story so there is a mental connection as well.

Once you are in that relaxed and connected frame of mind, reading together also allows you to open yourself up to your sexuality. This can happen in a couple of different ways. If the story you are reading includes some scenes of romance, your mind (and body) will naturally start to go to a sexier place. In addition, as you are lying together, one or both of you might also start to stroke your lover.

Having your mind partly focused on the story while also connecting physically ironically helps you to be more present in your body because you are short-circuiting your mental chatter. You just won't have the bandwidth to start narrating to yourself about insecurities and worries while you are also trying to follow the story, which frees your mind and body up to simply enjoy the caresses as they come. Many is the time we started to read to one another and had to literally throw the book down because our motors were revved up and ready to move on to Phase Two.

You may not be Jane Austen fans, but there are countless options out there for books you could read together that would engage your mind and body. You will want to keep this pretty light because your brain can only focus on so much while your body is warming up for fun and adventure. The key will be finding something you can both enjoy and that will include some scenes you will both find sexy. Alternatively, reading this book aloud together or other books about connecting sexually can be a great option.

A variation of reading to one another in bed would be to lie in bed together listening to an audio book. We highly recommend you at least give the reading version of this game a try first, however, because having to focus enough to do the reading can create its own form of sexual tension. As with many of the games we describe in putting the Play in Foreplay, there is something exciting about trying to stimulate your partner while also knowing you are not actually about to have sex. You have a job to do here, after all, and you better stick to the script! The sex will come if and when you are both ready, and the longer the build-up, the more glorious the release.

TALK CLEAN TO ME

It seems to be a sort of cliché in books and movies that people get turned on by talking dirty to one another. As we discussed in the section titled "What Do I Call It," however, the use of crude language is going to be a turn-off to many people—women in particular. And for many, having to say or hear those types of words will cause discomfort and a sense of internal shut down. Why not flip this idea on its head?

We invented a little game we call "Talk Clean to Me." In this game, one of you will play the narrator and will also take the more dominant role in caressing and kissing your partner as you relate your story. Unlike some of our other foreplay games, here your partner does not have to lay there exclusively receiving, but he will be the listener. The narrator's job is to create a warm, evocative and sensual fantasy. It is extremely helpful in this game if the two of you have taken the time first to discuss your nomenclature of choice for your respective genitals. This allows the narrator to use the very words his lover longs to hear in spinning their tale of bliss. You want to take your lover on a little fantasy adventure.

As an example, let's say your preferred terms are jade garden (for her) and wand of light (for him). The narrator might start by describing the trip you will be taking through a mystical garden by an ancient river. She might describe what things look like there, what sort of animal and bird life you encounter on your journey, and how everything takes on a phosphorescent glow when it is illuminated by her partner's magical wand of light. Near the garden is this turquoise bubbling steam and the two of you jump into it, feeling the soft cool water caressing your skin. You let the current take you on a gentle journey down the river to a distant shore where a warm soft sandy beach awaits. And on it goes from there…

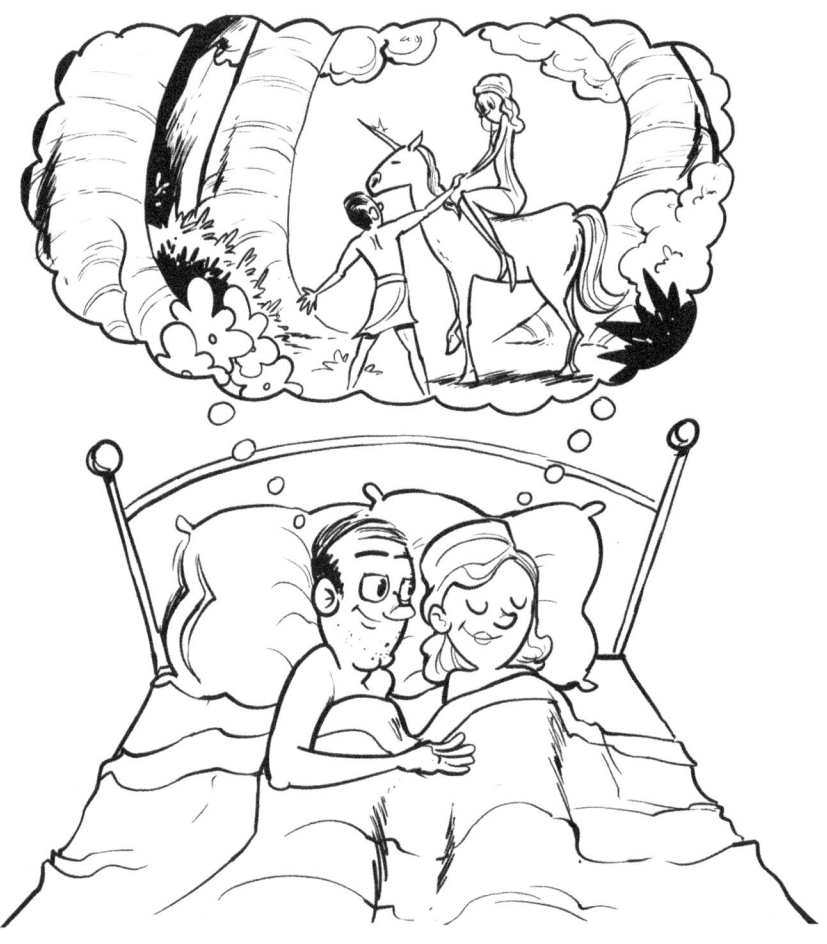

If you have a hard time making things up out of whole cloth, you might retell the story of a special day the two of you shared on a favorite vacation. Add in as many colorful details as you can think of to really put yourselves back in that place. Go through your senses for ideas. What was the quality of the light? What sorts of smells were present? Do you remember any delicious foods you enjoyed? What kinds of sounds could you hear? As with all of the other games we have described, the idea is to occupy your lover's mind enough to open it to pleasure by shutting down the mental chatter that otherwise might get in the way of connection.

BLINDFOLDS

All of our games have two things in common: they are designed to wake up the body and silence the mind's incessant chatter. We want to create sensations that feel new, exciting and surprising to help you stay present while also helping you to shut off your inner narrator so it won't sabotage your ability to Be Here Now.

One fun way to accomplish both is through the use of a blindfold. You will notice we make repeated references to this option as a way to kick many of our other games up a notch. Some great options for blindfolds include satiny sleep masks or a silky scarf tied gently but snuggly across your eyes.

The blindfold works on a variety of levels. First, it adds this element of surprise that makes every touch or kiss unexpected, which helps keep you very present in the moment. It also conjures up feelings of potential danger, which can heighten your senses and create some adrenaline, even though at a deeper level you know you are not actually at any risk of harm.

Dr. Ava Cadell, certified sex counselor and author of NeuroLoveology, notes that blindfolds can empower women and actually distract them from any hang-ups they may have with their bodies.

"It's even better for the ladies to blindfold their men, because that gives women more confidence," she said. "I've had so many clients that told me that once they blindfold their lover, they can do things and say things. They're ten times bolder than they've ever been. It liberates them."

As with all of our other suggestions, try it on for size and see what it feels like. Whether you are the blindfolded partner or the one controlling the action, blindfolds can be a great way to spice things up.

HEALTH

Even if you and your partner are committed to a better love life, and even if you've created the space and ability to "Be Here Now," serious medical or psychological issues can interfere with your enjoyment or even ability to have sex.

Vaginal pain and dryness, erectile difficulties, and loss of libido for both men and women may have medical causes that require professional help. The good news is that solutions are available for the vast majority of such issues, and we will describe some of these solutions in the sections below.

A great sex life does not generally spring from a dysfunctional relationship. Great sex requires the dropping of barriers and defenses of all kinds, not just your clothes. Dropping these defenses puts people, particularly women, into a very vulnerable position. Without love, kindness, and a deep mutual trust and respect it can be impossible to let go of these defenses. If there are real issues in your marriage or relationship these may need to be ironed out before you can get to the point of love and trust needed to foster a satisfying love life. Visit a psychologist or counselor who specializes in relationship issues. If the issues in your relationship are primarily around sex, professional sex therapists and counselors can help guide you back to a loving relationship.

The lesson here is that your problems have solutions. A mutually satisfying love life is one of the greatest gifts you can give one another, and worth the time and effort it takes. Find the solutions to your problems, and then go on the journey with us to "Be Here Now," and find your way to incendiary lovemaking. Stop and think for a moment about how your life and relationship would be with a fantastic and satisfying sex life. Isn't that worth your effort to make it come true?

DON'T BELIEVE ANY OF THIS

OK, here is the disclaimer. Neither of us are physicians or medical professionals of any kind. Julia gets sick at the sight of blood, although she did enjoy watching George Clooney on ER. Michael's last medical training was to learn CPR along with his daughters in preparation of them becoming babysitters. Considering our youngest is now in college, that was some time ago. None of this is meant to be medical advice. On all medical issues, consult a doctor, and if necessary, a specialist.

What we want to do is give you hope that a great sex life is possible. Many people find it embarrassing to even talk to their doctors about things like sexual pain, problems with erections, vaginal dryness or loss of libido. Many people live with these conditions for the rest of their lives, not knowing that for the vast majority of seniors, there are solutions. In this section we discuss common problems that affect your ability to have sex, and describe some of the solutions to these problems. Once you have the ability to have sex, all the rest of this book is about how to make that sex incendiary!

VAGINAL DRYNESS AND PAIN DURING SEX

Let's get one thing straight right at the start. You are completely normal. Loss of vaginal lubrication and experiencing some pain or irritation during intercourse is extremely common for post-menopausal women. You are not broken or deficient in any way, and your problems have solutions.

However, it's also possible you may not have a problem at all. As our bodies age, it generally takes more foreplay and romance to get the juices flowing, and you may not have a lack of lubrication but rather a lack of foreplay and a "Be Here Now" environment that allows you to focus on the sensations and romance. Also, if you have not had sex frequently in the last months or years, a problem with lubrication may work itself out as you enjoy sex more regularly, as regular sex promotes vaginal health and vaginal blood flow. However, here we will assume there is, at least temporarily, a problem with either lubrication or pain during intercourse.

The solutions to pain and vaginal dryness include everything from the simplest and easiest to those that require more medical supervision. Below we list some of these solutions in rough order of simple to complex.

If you are having mild vulvar discomfort or irritation, begin by avoiding certain soaps and scents. Use soft white unscented toilet paper. Wash your underwear in detergents without perfumes or dyes, and stop using fabric softeners or anti-cling products. Avoid using perfumed lotion, scented wipes, douches, or any other perfumed products on the inner vulva. And while we believe in cleanliness in sex, don't extend that to putting soap inside the inner vulva, as it can cause irritation. Just rinse your labia in the shower with warm water, using your fingers if needed to remove any excess discharge that may be hanging around.

The next solution is artificial vaginal lubricants, which are covered extensively in our "Arousal and Lubrication" and "All About Lubes" sections. A little slip-and-slide in you or on him can make all the difference.

But vaginal lubes are used only during sex, and there are other products that moisturize your vagina and vulva in the same way that you may moisturize your face and hands, and for the same reason, to promote and maintain soft supple skin. These products are not meant to be used during sex, but regularly as directed. In fact, it's better not to use them just before sex, especially if they include estrogen, as the estrogen can be absorbed into your partner's penis.

Vaginal moisturizers, unlike lubricants, are absorbed into the skin and cling to the vaginal walls, similar to natural secretions. Some moisturizers have an applicator to make it easy to put the moisturizer where it's needed most. Some of these products include K-Y Silk-E, Moist Again, Fresh Start, Luvens, K-Y Liquibeads, and Replens.

Another great solution, but one that you will need to get from your doctor, is low-dose vaginal estrogen in the form of either a cream, a tiny vaginal tablet, or a ring. These products have been around for 30 years, and have been found to restore vaginal blood flow, reverse thinning vaginal walls, and improve flexibility. They are remarkably effective, with up to 93 percent of women reporting significant improvement and 57 percent to 75 percent reporting that their sexual comfort is fully restored.

Available products include Estrace, Neo-Estrone, and Premarin creams, the Vagifem vaginal tablet, and Estring low dose vaginal ring, among others. Often, vaginal atrophy can respond more quickly to low-dose vaginal therapy than to higher dose hormone pills and patches.

You should use the lowest dose that is effective for you, and if you've had breast cancer or are at high risk for it, make sure you mention this to your doctor, so they can help you weigh the risks and benefits.

The creams are applied 2 to 3 times a week, the vaginal tablet inserted twice a week, and the low dose vaginal ring will be effective for 3 months before being taken out and replaced, and does not need to be removed for sex. Most women find the tablet or ring less messy than applying the cream. All forms of low-dose estrogen therapy are about the same in effect and have minimal side effects.

You can expect improvements to vaginal moisture and overall vaginal health within a few weeks, although severe vaginal atrophy may take some months to heal.

If you have been without sex for months or years, your pain may be related to your vagina atrophying and becoming too small for your partner's penis. There are vaginal dilators which will help you stretch and relax your vaginal walls to allow for more comfortable sex. These dildo-like dilators start about the width of your finger and graduate up to that of a fully-erect large penis. For your greatest comfort it is best to work up to one that is slightly larger than your partner's penis.

Finally, there are higher dose estrogen treatments that raise estrogen levels in the entire body via swallowed pills, patches or gels applied to the arm rather than locally as with low-dose vaginal estrogen therapy. These are generally prescribed for women with severe hot flashes or night sweats during menopause. You should carefully weigh the risks and benefits with your doctor, as some studies indicate that systemic hormone therapy may produce higher risks of heart attack, stroke, blood clots, and breast cancer, especially in older women.

ERECTILE DIFFICULTIES

We assume that you've heard about Erectile Dysfunction (ED). It would be hard not to hear about it, as our email junk boxes fill with badly spelled Viagra ads, and our TV often features Bob Dole or handsome couples with dreamy, satisfied smiles touting the latest ED drug. (Why are these couples always in weird places like side-by-side bathtubs outdoors??)

These ads are so prevalent, you might think that every man over 30 in America has ED. Do you have ED? Well, maybe, and maybe not.

If you suffer an occasional penis vacation day, or find that you wax and wane a bit during sex, or maybe that your erection isn't as rock-hard as you remember, that's not Erectile Dysfunction, but just the effects of growing older. See "You Are Not Your Penis" and the "How to Have an Erection After 50" sections. In those sections we talk about many things you can do without drugs to improve your blood flow and reduce your out-of-service hours.

But if, sober and healthy, you regularly can't get at least moderately stiff after extended foreplay or masturbation, you should consult your doctor. You are certainly not alone. University of Chicago researchers found that among men aged 50 to 64, about one-third suffered ED, with the percentage rising to 44 percent for men aged 65 to 85.

An important reason to talk to your doctor, regardless of whether you would like an ED drug prescription, is that ED is often just a by-product of other health issues which may need addressing, and in many cases, addressing the underlying health issue may solve your ED problem anyway.

Common health issues that can affect your ability to "rise to the occasion" include:

- Diabetes
- Obesity
- Heart disease
- High blood pressure
- High cholesterol
- Depression
- Low testosterone
- Enlarged prostate
- Sleep apnea
- Multiple sclerosis
- Parkinson's disease

Also, common medications can affect your erections. You could speak to your doctor about using alternate medications that would not have as much of a sexual side effect, or if that is not possible, going on a lower dose of your medication. Medications that can have sexual side effects such as ED include:

- Antihistamines
- Calcium blockers
- Hormone therapy
- Blood pressure medicine
- Enlarged prostate medication
- Antidepressants

ED drugs work well for about two thirds of all men with Erectile Dysfunction. While you've certainly heard of Viagra, Cialis is actually more common, primarily because it's effects last 24 hours or more, as opposed to 4 to 6 hours typical for Viagra. (Don't worry. We don't mean the erection will last 24 hours, just your ability to have one!) Aside from Viagra and Cialis there is Levitra and a host of new drugs coming on the market. Since they may have different effects for different people, if one drug doesn't work, try another before giving up on ED drugs.

If ED drugs don't work or chronic health issues get in the way, your doctor, or a specialist, may have more options for you, up to and including penile implants. If none of that appeals to you or works for you, that does not mean the end of your sex life. Most men can have a full orgasm without being hard, and of course can sexually satisfy their partner without an erect penis.

LOSS OF LIBIDO IN WOMEN

Libido or sexual desire comes in two flavors. Remember when you just "had to have it"? When the touch of a lover or even the thought of him moistened your panties and made your heart race? When you'd make love in a frenzy in the park in the dark, in his van, maybe standing pressed against a wall?

That form of libido or sexual desire was the "Need to have it" variety. Your body was producing the ultimate designer drugs, hormones that were refined by nature over millions of years to act on your subconscious to drive you to the sexual act for the purpose of procreation. Hormones work on the subconscious, not the conscious, so we are able to fool Mother Nature when we consciously prevented procreation through condoms or birth control pills. Even though procreation wasn't possible, the hormones still did their job by making you "Need it."

With menopause, the dealer supplying you those designer drugs has gone out of business. Without those specialized hormones and the subconscious desires they drove, female libido as a senior is no longer a "Need to have it" thing but a "Want to have it" thing.

Why would you "Want to have it"? Female libido has always been more complicated and more fragile than male libido, and much of this book is meant to remove the distractions and provide the environment where desire can flourish. However, if we feel pain during sex, through vaginal dryness and much thinner vaginal walls, or other physical pain such as arthritis, then wanting to have it becomes difficult. After all, you might even stop loving chocolate if every time you reached for a piece someone smacked you on the side of your head, right?

So first, if you are having pain during sex, find solutions, some of which are outlined in the "Vaginal Dryness and Pain During Sex" section, and create the physical and mental environment for sexual desire to flourish, as outlined in much of this book. One of the main tenets of this book is that once you've experienced regular "Incendiary" sex and awakened your body to it, then "Wanting it" becomes easier, because who wouldn't want steamy heat and mind-blowing orgasms now and then?

But also, there are treatments today that can get blood moving to the softer parts and give you a bit more of that "Need it" drive you used to have, and science is constantly searching for new and better treatments. In the following we will outline some of those treatments, starting with what you get over the counter, followed by treatments approved by the FDA, and finally treatments that have some proven effectiveness but are often prescribed "off-label" by competent physicians.

<u>Cannabis.</u> The first and best over-the-counter treatment that we know about is, yes, legal cannabis! Whether this actually directly improves sexual desire, or provides the environment for it to sprout, we can testify that for at least some people this increases sexual desire. Effects vary from person to person, and the wrong strain or wrong dosage can actually depress libido, but used correctly it can be magical. See all the sections under "Sex and Cannabis."

Warming Lubricants. While most lubricants are intended to address vaginal dryness during sex, another class of lubricants are "warming" lubricants designed to enhance sexual response. These lubricants cause warming or cooling sensations by using ingredients such as capsaicin (yes, the chemical that puts the "hot" in hot sauce!), menthol or primrose oil. Zestra, which uses primrose oil, was found to increase sexual response in a small research study.[11]

However, we would suggest you approach these with caution. Certainly some women have found these warming or cooling lubricants to be effective. However our experience with it was "Ouch!" Try just a very small amount at the beginning to assure that you can handle it, and have warm washcloths at the ready in case you feel like a wasp is stinging your most precious parts. As with fragrances, many women's vulvas are just too sensitive to tolerate ingredients like capsaicin or menthol.

Herbal Remedies. The internet is replete with herbal and "natural" products that claim to improve men's and women's sexual performance and satisfaction. These supplements, teas and creams are not regulated by the US Food and Drug Administration, and most have not been well studied, or shown clearly to provide the claimed sexual performance enhancement.

A small study seemed to show that a supplement called ArginMax, made from gingko, ginseng, damiana, vitamins, calcium, iron, selenium and zinc may boost libido, but it is probably too early to say that this

---

[11] https://www.businesswire.com/news/home/20050509005976/en/Zestra----Clinically-Proven-Arousal-Solution-Women

supplement clearly does improve performance. It's important to note that "herbal" and "natural" does not mean harmless. If you do use supplements of this kind, be sure to tell your doctor, so that they can evaluate any potential interactions you might have with other medications or conditions.

Female Viagra. Have you heard about "Female Viagra," the "Pink Pill"? Those are the names that news articles coined for the drug Flibanserin, brand named Addyi, a once-daily pill to improve female sexual dysfunction approved by the FDA in 2015. The original FDA approval was for pre-menopausal women only, but a 2014 study of 900 postmenopausal women with low sexual desire showed Flibanserin effective compared to placebos.[12] Like any drug, there can be side effects and it will not work for everyone, but the general efficacy seems well proven. The initial FDA trials included over 11,000 women, compared to the 3,000 men included in the original FDA Viagra trials.

One reason this may not be talk among your friends and family is that the current cost is reported to be high—as much as $800 per month. However, don't panic, this cost may reduce substantially in the near future, because Flibanserin can be produced as a generic starting in August of 2020.

Clitoral Vacuum. A clitoral therapy device has been approved by both the US FDA and Canadian governments to treat low sexual desire and arousal. The product is brand named Eros-CTD, a small vacuum pump that fits over your clitoris and uses suction to bring blood into the

---

[12] https://www.ncbi.nlm.nih.gov/pmc/articles/PMC5644557/

clitoris. The device requires a prescription in the US, but can be bought over the counter in Canada.

Bupropion (Wellbutrin). SSRI antidepressants (selective serotonin reuptake inhibitors) reduce sexual desire and response in some patients who take them for depression and anxiety. However, the antidepressant bupropion (Wellbutrin) is not an SSRI and works in a different manner. A small study that provided Wellbutrin to non-depressed women and men with desire and arousal difficulties was found to improve sexual functioning compared with a placebo.[13] While the finding is interesting, more study is required before bupropion is prescribed for treating lack of sexual desire. However, if you are on an SSRI, you could speak to your doctor about the possibility of switching to Wellbutrin, as at a minimum it does not have the negative sexual effects of SSRI's.

Testosterone. It is believed that extremely low levels of testosterone may contribute to reduced libido and weaker orgasmic response in some women. Many companies and researchers are studying whether testosterone therapy could be a safe and effective treatment for lack of sexual desire in women. A study among selected postmenopausal women with low sexual desire showed that testosterone delivered by a skin patch increased sexual desire and the frequency of satisfying sex among about 50 percent of participants.[14]

Testosterone is a hormone found in men, but is also produced in smaller amounts in women, particularly in the ovaries. Testosterone is necessary for muscle tone, a healthy sexual desire, and strong bones.

---
[13] http://journals.sagepub.com/doi/full/10.1177/2045125316629071
[14] https://www.nejm.org/doi/pdf/10.1056/nejmoa0707302

Testosterone in women decreases substantially during menopause, and often actually begins decreasing years before menopause. Women with very low testosterone levels may experience fatigue, depression, weight gain, muscle loss, and cognitive dysfunction along with dramatically decreased libido. (Ain't aging grand?)

While no testosterone products have been approved for sexual problems in women in the US or Canada, the testosterone patch has been approved in Europe for treating low sexual desire associated with surgically menopausal women. In the US, testosterone products in the form of skin patches, topical gels, sprays, or subcutaneous pellets are sometimes prescribed off-label to women.

Common side effects include acne and increased facial and body hair. Rare effects seen with high doses of testosterone might include permanent deepening of the voice, weight gain, liver problems, and enlargement of the clitoris.

Testosterone is converted to estrogen in the blood, and so some experts think that testosterone therapy might have some of the long-term risks associated with systemic estrogen therapy, including increased risk of breast cancer or heart disease. However this has not been proven.

Testosterone products for men, such as Androderm, Testoderm, and Androgel are prescribed to men in doses that are inappropriate for women, although these same products may be prescribed off-label for women at doses of one tenth of that provided for men.

DHEA. A Canadian clinical trial in postmenopausal women found that an intravaginal tablet containing DHEA improved all aspects of female sexual function, including desire, arousal, orgasm, and pain compared to the placebo. DHEA may hold promise as a safe and effective therapy for sexual problems in postmenopausal women, but more study is needed.

LOSS OF LIBIDO IN MEN

While loss of libido is less common in men than in women, a variety of chronic illnesses and other medical problems can reduce a man's sex drive. While erectile dysfunction (ED) does not directly cause a loss of libido, the psychological issues of not being able to achieve an erection can cause men to avoid sex. This is unfortunate, as most cases of erectile dysfunction can be treated. (See our section on "Erection Difficulties.") Any medical condition that interferes with blood flow can lead to difficulty maintaining an erection. Cardiovascular disease, hypertension, and diabetes can reduce blood flow to the body, including the genitals. Chronic alcoholism and even occasional excessive alcohol bingeing are well known to both inflame desire and reduce your ability to perform.

However, some men do suffer a loss of desire. Serious illnesses such as cancer will often dampen any thoughts of sex, as your body conserves its resources to fight the illness. Conditions such as thyroid disorders and tumors of the pituitary gland, which controls sex hormone production, can also lower libido.

A loss of desire can be related to hormones, particularly testosterone, and if you suffer from a reduced libido, getting your testosterone checked is a good idea. Certain illnesses, such as diabetes, have the effect of reducing testosterone. According to the American Diabetes Association, a man with type 2 diabetes is twice as likely to have low testosterone compared to a man who does not have diabetes. However, don't assume any loss of desire is related to a lack of testosterone. Medical experts are concerned that many men are being treated for low testosterone who do not need it, and so suffer unnecessarily from the side effects of such treatments.

Depression may also reduce your desire for sex, along with your desire for everything else in life. Taking antidepressants may help with the symptoms of depression, but the most common antidepressants are SSRIs (selective serotonin reuptake inhibitors), which can reduce sexual desire and response in patients who take them. The antidepressant bupropion (Wellbutrin) is not an SSRI and works in a different manner. A small study that provided Wellbutrin to non-depressed women and men with desire and arousal difficulties was found to improve sexual functioning compared with a placebo. While more study is required before Wellbutrin is prescribed to non-depressed people for lack of libido, if you suffer from depression and are on an SSRI, you could speak to your doctor about the possibility of switching to Wellbutrin, as Wellbutrin does not have the negative sexual effects of SSRIs.

Finally, a number of prescription drugs have side effects of lowering libido, including common blood pressure drugs. If you think this may be a cause of your reduced sex drive, talk to your doctor about lowering your dosage or switching to alternative medicines without sexual side effects.

SEX THERAPY AND COUNSELING

Issues such as low libido and erectile dysfunction may have an emotional or psychological component, and so sex therapy or psychological counseling may be helpful. Several studies have shown that drug therapy combined with sex therapy or counseling can work better than drugs alone at bringing sex back into your life.

In addition, mutually satisfying sex is more than just erections and lubrication. The quality of your relationship, and the emotional baggage that one or both of you may be carrying due to lack of regular sex, can lie at the root of loss of libido. If your relationship or psychological problems cannot be cured with our suggestions under our "It's Been a Loooong Time" section, consider a counselor or sex therapist.

To find therapists who specialize in sexual issues, visit the American Association of Sexuality Educators, Counselors, and Therapists (https://www.aasect.org/), the Society for Sex Therapy and Research (https://sstarnet.org/), or the American Board of Sexology (http://theamericanboardofsexology.com/).

RESOURCES

Websites change, as does the quality of the companies they advertise. As always, do your own research. If you find a bad link, please contact us at www.incendiarysex.com.

Sex Stores

- www.yelp.com – Search for "adult sex stores"

Sex Toys

- www.we-vibe.com
- www.lelo.com
- www.jimmyjane.com
- www.jejoue.com
- www.womanizer.com

Lube

- www.cheaplubes.com

Cannabis

- www.leafly.com – Dispensary locations and information
- www.foira.com – Cannabis infused sex lube

Safe Sex

- www.plannedparenthood.org/learn/stds-hiv-safer-sex/safer-sex

Sexual Counseling

- www.aasect.org - The American Association of Sexuality Educators, Counselors, and Therapists
- www.sstarnet.org - The Society for Sex Therapy and Research
- www.theamericanboardofsexology.com - The American Board of Sexology

Sexual Health

- www.ashasexualhealth.org – The American Sexual Health Organization

Additional Reading

- *Come As You Are* by Dr. Emily Nagoski
- *Vagina, A New Biography*, by Naomi Wolf
- *Tanta, the Art of Conscious Loving*, by Charles and Caroline Muir
- *The Science of Trust*, by John Gottman

APPENDIX: EROTIC GUIDED MASSAGE SCRIPT

The following is our suggested script for you to use when recording your own guided sensual massage. Think of this as a starting place. Give it a try and see what works for you and what doesn't, and refine as needed. Simply read the script, slowly and sexily and with the appropriate pauses into a recording device like your smartphone, and then play it back for both of you via a blue tooth speaker, and enjoy an erotic massage experience. What a great gift to give your lover, letting them know how much you care about their pleasure. You may find, as we did, that just making the guided massage audio and imagining it as you go can be a stimulating experience on its own.

A guided massage should always begin by creating the space to "Be Here Now," so see all the sections under "Be Here Now." Since you will want massage oil for this, check our tip for having hot oil at the ready under the "Ready and Waiting" section. Note that the "pauses" we suggest are not pauses to the massage, but to give you time to do the moves that the script is suggesting before moving on to the next technique.

In the following script, the text in quotation marks is to be read, while text in parenthesis is for information only. Feel free to adapt this to your own style, to add or modify any bit of it. You can put a musical sound track directly into your guided massage, or you can just have music playing in the background from some other device while you enjoy the guided massage. Assuming you pause about 20 seconds on the "Short Pauses" below, then the entire massage will last about 40 to 45 minutes. If you want a shorter version, concentrate on the lower back, buttocks and thighs. Deep massage and relaxation in these areas, with rocking of the legs and pelvis, is the quickest way to encourage blood flow and build erotic energy.

One final note: Don't take this too seriously. If you don't like a certain bit as you are giving or receiving the massage, do something else until the next instruction comes along. If you and your partner get fully aroused part way through, don't feel obligated to finish the massage. We ourselves rarely make it all the way to the end—for very happy reasons.

The Guided Massage Script

"Take a few moments to connect with your partner. Stop and touch each other. Breath together. One partner can spoon the other, or you can look into each other's eyes and breath together, letting go of all the stress of the day, leaving the stress outside of you before you start your massage."

(Pause 1-2 minutes)

"Now, gently ask your partner to lie face down on the bed and invite them to get comfortable, close their eyes if they want to, and relax themselves into the softness."

(Pause 10 seconds)

"Begin by entering into physical touch together. Stroke and touch your partner lightly on all parts of their body. Focus on your touch. Bring all your sensitivity and awareness into your touch. Breath calmness through your fingertips into your partners skin."

(Pause 1 minute)

"Begin by massaging the scalp. Gently place your fingertips along the hairline at the base of the skull. Make small circles with a firm pressure or to your partner's liking. Slowly work your fingers up your partner's scalp and slowly sift your fingers through your partner's hair."

(Short pause)

"Take a good amount of hair into your hand and gently pull with a slow but firm pressure. Make sure you take enough hair in hand, because pulling on small strands is not pleasurable. Ask your partner if they would like you to pull lighter or harder."

(Pause 1 minute)

"Ask your partner if it is okay if you straddle their butt. If that is uncomfortable you could kneel or stand to the side of their head."

(Pause 10 seconds)

"Now, take your fingertips and lightly tease along the area at the back of the head where the neck meets the skull. The back of the neck and near the hairline is an erogenous zone. Perhaps you will want to breath into the back of your partner's neck or lightly kiss or lick the area to awaken the sensations."

(Short pause)

"Next, use your thumbs at the base of the skull to feel around for any tiny indentations. Massaging these little pockets can be very relaxing, as there are many muscles that attach in this area. Press your thumbs into the indentations at the base of the skull and make very small circles. Ask your partner if they would like this firmer or gentler."

(Pause 1 minute)

"To further relax your partner try squeezing the muscles of the back of the neck. Squeeze and release, squeeze and release as you work along the deeper muscles in the back and sides of their neck. You can use one or both of your hands. Breath relaxation into your partner with your hands. The deeper you relax your partner, the more arousal can build. Deep relaxation allows more oxygenated blood and helps build arousal. Ask your partner to breathe deeply and release all their tension with each breath."

(Short pause)

"Now, if you aren't already using massage oil, this is a good time to do so, as the next techniques can be uncomfortable with dry hands. Drizzle oil across your partner's back and sensuously smooth it in. If the oil is already hot, drizzle it directly onto their back. If not, warm the oil up in your hands before smoothing it onto your partner. If you are straddling your partner's butt, you can add an extra level of arousal by sensuously circling your pelvis against their butt. Check in with your partner to see how this feels to them."

(Pause 1 minute)

"Place your palms on their sacrum, the triangular bone at the base of the spine. Firmly press the heels of your hands into the muscles alongside the spine and push up toward the shoulders. Once you are there, drag your hands back down their sides. Add warm oil as necessary to create a smooth and erogenous touch. Invite your partner to breathe deeply. Check with your partner about whether they'd like it firmer or gentler."

(Pause 1 minute)

"Work the muscles along your partner's shoulders. Squeeze and release, squeeze and release. If you'd like, press your chest down on their back, breath into their hair and kiss or lick as you or your partner like."

(Pause 1 minute)

"Work the muscles along the spine. Press your forefingers or thumbs along each side of the spine and slide firmly up from sacrum to shoulders. Press your forefingers or thumbs along the edge of your partner's shoulder bones. These areas hold a lot of stress. For a deeper massage you can kneel at your partner's side and press your elbow into the large muscles of your partner's lower back, and slowly move it up alongside the spine. Be careful not to press hard directly over the spine."

(Pause 1 minute)

"Now, move so that your kneeling or standing at your partner's head and reverse this technique by pushing your hands down, pushing down from shoulders to sacrum alongside the spine. This will give a nice stretch to your partner's back."

(Pause 1 minute)

"To finish off the back massage, spread your fingers wide, just barely touching the skin. And as lightly as you can, slowly work your way up your partner's back, like the brushing of butterfly wings. Build erotic energy by bringing your lips down so they are almost but not quite touching your partner's skin. Gently breathe or blow hot air onto the spots you think need a little more attention. Many people find this light touch after a firm massage very pleasurable."

(Pause 1 minute)

"Now, standing or kneeling by your partner's side, place both hands on the far side of the rib cage and pull up as if you are trying to lift it off the mattress. Alternate your hands one after the other as you glide up your partner's side pulling gently and lifting. This will help to open up your partner's breathing and lead to deep relaxation."

(Short pause)

"When you have done a few repetitions on one side of the rib cage move on to the other side and stroke and lift."

(Short pause)

"To ease any remaining tension in the lower back, you can drum your fingertips on the sacrum, or use the sides of your hand or loose fists to gently pound. Check in with your partner on whether they want it harder or gentler. You may be surprised at how much pressure they can take in this spot."

(Short pause)

"Now, place your palms sideways on the sacrum and rock the sacrum back and forth, rocking your partner's body back and forth. This can be greatly relaxing. Ask your partner if they would like it slower or faster."

(Short pause)

"Kneading and massaging your partner's buttocks and the back of their thighs is one of the best ways to release tension and bring blood flow to the genitals. Rocking your partner's pelvis and butt back and forth will build more and more sexual energy."

(Pause 10 seconds)

"Place cupped hands on one butt cheek and push your hands towards one another while pressing into the butt cheek in a sliding and kneading motion, back and forth, alternating hands."

(Short pause)

"When you have fully relaxed one butt cheek, move on to the other side."

(Short pause)

"Using both hands, push the butt cheeks together, and then apart. Push one cheek up and the other down, then reverse."

(Short pause)

"Reach your hands to far side of the hip and pull up gently, sliding your hand up and rocking the pelvis. Alternate hands, pulling first up with one then the other."

(Short pause)

"When you've done a few strokes on one side, go to the other side and pull up and rock the pelvis gently."

(Short pause)

"Starting with the far side of the hips, scratch your fingers gently across the hip and across your partner's bottom. This light scratching may excite sexual energy."

(Short pause)

"Now, straddle your partner's thighs. Press down and massage the buttocks with the heels of your hands. You may find indentations in the muscles of your partners buttocks. Press and massage these indentations firmly, making little circles over the spots. Press and massage the tailbone and the little pockets around the tailbone. Check in with your partner about how this feels to them."

(Pause 1 minute)

"Perhaps the greatest erogenous zone that few people know about is the gluteal fold, the crease at the bottom of each butt cheek where it meets the leg. Using the pads of both thumbs push into both creases until you feel a bony structure underneath. Press here, and then begin deeply massaging in small circles."

(Pause 1-2 minutes)

"To build even more arousal, lightly stroke your thumb pads or fingertips along the gluteal fold. If you'd like, bend down and add your breath, licks and kisses to further activate the sexual energy."

(Short pause)

"Now, straddle your partner's calves, and, with plenty of oil, push and knead with both hands up one thigh all the way to the buttocks. Squeeze and knead the muscles of the back of the thigh. Rock the leg side to side if you'd like. This rocking will produce a pleasurable rubbing sensation in the genital area that can be very arousing to your partner."

(Pause 30 seconds)

"After you've finished one thigh, switch to the other thigh. Have your partner breathe deep and relax and stretch as you massage the thighs."

(Pause 30 seconds)

"Switch now to a softer touch, lightly tracing your fingertips along the back of the knee and the back of the thigh, using a slightly scratching, featherlight touch not only up the back of the thighs, but across the buttocks as well."

(Short pause)

"It's time to move to the other side of the body, but before you do, give this side of your partner's body a fond but temporary farewell. Softly caress your hands up your partner's body, sliding over thighs and buttocks, back and neck. Kissing, licking and blowing lightly is encouraged. Lay your entire body briefly over your partner's, and massage them with your whole body."

(Pause 1 minute)

"Now, softly ask your partner to slowly turn so that he or she is lying face up."

(Pause 10 seconds)

"Standing or kneeling at your partner's side, start now by caressing the face with two fingertips from each hand stroking from the center of your partner's forehead out to the temples. Once you have done a few strokes, do the same to your partner's chin, starting in the center and smoothing out along the jawline."

(Short pause)

"Massage the temples by placing your finger tips on both sides and gently jiggling your hands back and forth to send vibrations through them. Then make small circles and invite your partner to breathe deeply."

(Short pause)

"Allow yourself a little play. Trace the outer edge of your partner's ears with your fingertips. Breathe into the neck and ears if your partner likes that. Lightly squeeze the earlobes and gently pull them down and out. Gently trace your partner's lips with your fingertips or tongue."

(Pause 1 minute)

"Massage your partner's arm, squeezing and kneading the muscles from the shoulder to the fingers. Intertwine your fingers with your partner's, sliding and massaging the fingers as you do so. Massage the inside of your partner's palms, pressing deeply at the center of the palm and the base of the thumb."
(Pause 30 seconds)

"When you've finished one arm, massage the other arm, not forgetting your partner's palm and fingers."

(Pause 30 seconds)

"Now lightly stroke your fingertips or fingernails down both arms, including the insides of the elbows. Kissing, tasting, and licking are often appreciated as well."

(Short pause)

"For the chest massage you can stay at your partner's side, or for an extra level of arousal you could straddle them genital to genital. Begin with a hand resting on your partner's sternum which is at the center of the chest. Rest there for a moment, both you and your partner breathing deeply. Now stroke your hands between the breasts and circle around them, slowly spiraling in towards the nipples, but without touching them."

(Short pause)

"Cup the breasts or pectorals in your hands. Rotate them gently around, up and down. Spread them apart and gently back together. Be creative here. Some people love having their nipples pinched and pulled lightly, others don't. If your partner likes their nipples touched, stroke the nipples with the palms of your hands, rotating slowing. Follow that with a light scratching of the nipples with your fingertips. Squeeze the nipples between thumb and forefinger and gently pull while your partner breathes in. Or if your partner would not enjoy this sort of stimulation, you can kiss and caress the entire chest, stroking along the side of the chest and the breasts. Kiss and blow on the parts that need more attention."

(Pause 1 minute)

"Now, with plenty of oil, stroke the abdomen in a circular motion, massaging gently."

(Short pause)

"Another wonderful erogenous zone is located from below the belly button to the top of the pubis. Stroke the area in a circular motion, and gently pull up, stretching the pubis area a little. Then, start at the center and stroke to the outside with both hands."

(Short pause)

"Take your partner's hips in your hand and gently rock the pelvis back and forth. Alternate between rocking the pelvis and stroking the abdomen."

(Short pause)

"Next, take your hands and lightly stroke from your partner's hips down the outside of one leg all the way to the feet, and then start again at the pubis and stroke the inner thigh down to the feet."

(Short pause)

"When you have finished one leg, lightly stroke and massage the other one."

(Short pause)

"Now, massage your partner's foot. Pressing into the bottom of the foot activates and stimulates sexual energy that your partner may feel deep inside. Press deeply with your thumbs into the bottom of the foot. Press the pads at the base of the toes. Gently squeeze each toe in turn, massaging the sensitive sides of the toes. Sucking and licking the toes can be erotic for many people. If you are a woman, pressing your breasts and nipples into his toes can be enjoyable."

(Pause 30 seconds)

"When you've done one foot, move to the other. Pressing, squeezing, licking."

(Pause 30 seconds)

"Now, close out the front massage as you did for your partner's back massage. Softly caress your hands up your partner's body, sliding over thighs and the area from pubis to navel, their chest or breasts, their sides, back and neck. Kissing, licking and blowing lightly is encouraged. Lay your entire body over your partner's, and massage them with your whole body, and kiss their lips, ears and neck."

(Pause 1 minute)

"While the massage is over, the evening is not. No need to rush. You may want to hold each other, and look into each other's eyes, or just enjoy the feeling of total relaxation. If lovemaking is an option, you can begin by slowly kissing and caressing and move on to a genital massage or other pleasures. Be sure to thank your partner for joining you in this relaxing and pleasurable experience."

AFTERWORD - MICHAEL

Writing this book has been a real joy. We hope that you will find at least some of our tips and suggestions useful, and that you and your partner will share some of the deep love, emotional closeness, and out-of-this-world amazing sex that Julia and I have found.

In closing, here is one final tip for having amazing, incendiary sex: Write a sex book with your wife! I say, "Julia, baby, you sweet thing. I think it's time for some more book research!"

AFTERWORD – JULIA

We started this project as a bit of a lark, trying to come up with something we could do together as a team. We had no idea where it might lead. There were many unexpected benefits to this process. One of those was the way I now think of myself. In addition to all the other roles and labels I had (wife, mother, working professional, etc.) I now had "sexpert" to add to my list. Sometimes just a small shift in thinking can have a huge impact.

Seeing myself as a sexy person and someone who is willing to stretch my boundaries to expand my enjoyment of sex has allowed me to fulfill that destiny. I encourage anyone reading this book to expand their own sense of identity as well. You are sexy. You deserve to have great sex. And your partner deserves to go on this crazy wild journey with you.

Made in the USA
Coppell, TX
12 January 2025

44308619R00134